Textbook of Conventional Fixed Partial Dentures

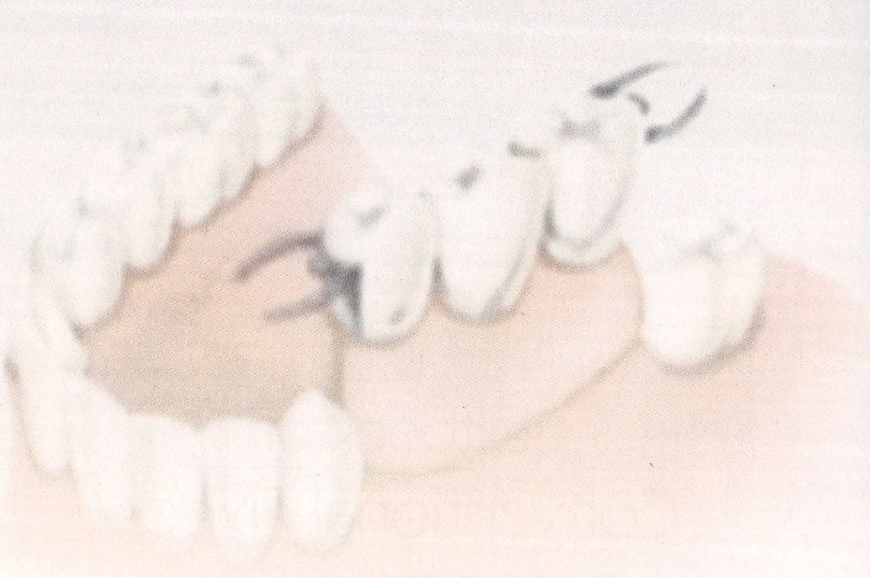

Textbook of Conventional Fixed Partial Dentures

Reshma Prabhu
MDS (prosthodontics and implantology)
Consultant Prosthodontist and Implantologist

CBS Publishers & Distributors Pvt Ltd

New Delhi • Bengaluru • Chennai • Kochi • Mumbai • Pune
Hyderabad • Kolkata • Nagpur • Patna • Vijayawada

Disclaimer

Science and technology are constantly changing fields. New research and experience broaden the scope of information and knowledge. The author has tried her best in giving information available to her while preparing the material for this book. Although, all efforts have been made to ensure optimum accuracy of the material, yet it is quite possible some errors might have been left uncorrected. The publisher, the printer and the author will not be held responsible for any inadvertent errors, omissions or inaccuracies.

Textbook of
Conventional Fixed Partial Dentures

ISBN: 978-81-239-2360-4

First Edition: 2014

Published by Satish Kumar Jain for
CBS Publishers & Distributors Pvt Ltd
4819/XI Prahlad Street, 24 Ansari Road, Daryaganj, New Delhi 110 002, India.
Ph: 23289259, 23266861, 23266867 Website: www.cbspd.com
Fax: 011-23243014 e-mail: delhi@cbspd.com; cbspubs@airtelmail.in.
Corporate Office : 204 FIE, Industrial Area, Patparganj, Delhi 110 092
Ph: 4934 4934 Fax: 4934 4935 e-mail: publishing@cbspd.com; publicity@cbspd.com

Branches

- **Bengaluru:** Seema House 2975, 17th Cross, K.R. Road, Banasankari 2nd Stage, Bengaluru 560 070, Karnataka
  Ph: +91-80-26771678/79 Fax: +91-80-26771680 e-mail: bangalore@cbspd.com
- **Chennai:** 20, West Park Road, Shenoy Nagar, Chennai 600 030, Tamil Nadu
  Ph: +91-44-26260666, 26208620 Fax: +91-44-42032115 e-mail: chennai@cbspd.com
- **Kochi:** 36/14 Kalluvilakam, Lissie Hospital Road, Kochi 682 018, Kerala
  Ph: +91-484-4059061-65 Fax: +91-484-4059065 e-mail: kochi@cbspd.com
- **Mumbai:** 83-C, Dr E Moses Road, Worli, Mumbai-400018, Maharashtra
  Ph: +91-9833017933 e-mail: mumbai@cbspd.com
- **Pune:** Bhuruk Prestige, Sr. No. 52/12/2+1+3/2 Narhe, Haveli (Near Katraj-Dehu Road Bypass), Pune 411 041, Maharashtra
  Ph: +91-20-64704058, 64704059, 32392277 Fax: +91-20-24300160 e-mail: pune@cbspd.com

Representatives

- **Hyderabad** 0-9885175004
- **Nagpur** 0-9021734563
- **Vijayawada** 0-9000660880
- **Kolkata** 0-9831437309, 0-9051152362
- **Patna** 0-9334159340

Printed at : R P Printers, Noida

Preface

Fixed prosthodontics is the art and science of replacing missing tooth structure in a single tooth or replacing missing teeth with a prosthesis. That said, the treatment should be directed at achieving a healthy mouth and attaining this requires a combination of many aspects of dental treatment. The right treatment begins with patient education that is directed not only at maintenance of the given prosthesis but also at prevention of progress of existing disease or occurrence of new disease. This is followed by a sound diagnosis, adequate periodontal and operative treatments, evaluation of the final occlusion and regular follow-up, maintenance appointments. This sequence when followed will help attain the goals of the planned treatment.

This textbook is designed as a guide for a learner, postgraduate student or an experienced practitioner alike. The book is divided into four parts: Each part contains chapters that are descriptive of the heading. Part I introduces the student to the branches of prosthodontics, various definitions and the basics of other specialties closely associated with fixed prosthodontics. Part II gives a detailed description of the parts of a fixed partial denture (FPD). The clinical procedures with a short description of materials used in each procedure are discussed in Part III while procedures closely associated with the clinical procedures and failures of treatment are described in Part IV.

An attempt has been made to give a comprehensive knowledge about the subject. However, no textbook can cover all topics entirely. For an in-depth knowledge about dental materials, periodontics, endodontics, occlusion and laboratory techniques, it is recommended that the students refer to the standard textbooks of the respective subjects.

Reshma Prabhu

Acknowledgements

This book is the result of many invisible hands that have helped me in its preparation and presentation. This work would not have been possible without the continuous support and encouragement of my family, colleagues and students. Many people have indirectly contributed for the completion of this book. However, I would like to extend a special acknowledgement to Dr Sarandha DL, Professor, Department of Prosthodontics, for her guidance in compiling the text. My sincere thanks to Dr Sunil S, Associate Professor, Department of Periodontics, for his contribution of clinical pictures of periodontal surgeries. This book is dedicated to my family whose patience and continuous support has been the motivation for its completion.

Reshma Prabhu

Contents

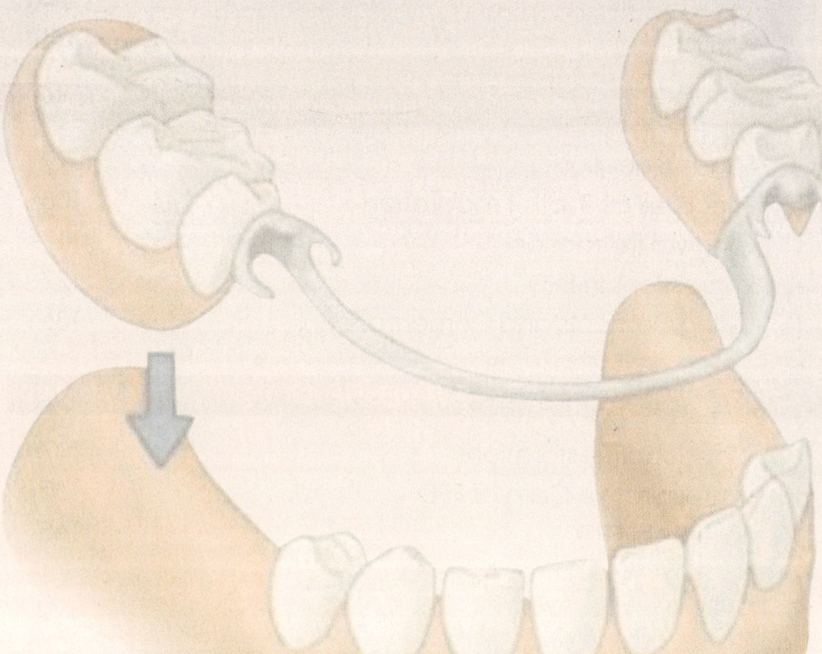

PART I

Introductory Chapters

1

Introduction

Dentistry is the health science that is involved in the evaluation, diagnosis, prevention, and surgical or non-surgical treatment of diseases, disorders and conditions of the oral cavity, maxillofacial area and the adjacent and associated structures, masticatory muscles and their impact on the human body. Complete oral health is an essential part of overall health. An esthetic quality of the mouth, its restoration or simply its enhancement is finding a permanent place in the practice of dentistry.

The scope of fixed prosthodontics ranges from restoration or replacement of a single tooth to replacement of entire arch. The fixed prosthodontic treatment like other prosthodontic treatments is aimed at improving the patient comfort and masticatory ability, maintains the health and integrity of the dental arches and has the added benefit of being secured to the teeth or implants. This, in many cases, adds to the confidence and self-image of the patient.

Branches of Prosthodontics

I. Removable prosthodontics: (a) Complete and (b) Partial
II. Fixed prosthodontics
III. Maxillofacial prosthodontics
IV. Implant prosthodontics

Definition of Terms (From GPT 2005)

Prosthodontics is the dental specialty pertaining to the diagnosis, treatment planning, rehabilitation and maintenance of the oral function, comfort, appearance and health of the patients with clinical conditions associated with missing or deficient teeth and/or maxillofacial tissues using biocompatible substitutes.

Fixed Prosthodontics: The branch of prosthodontics concerned with the replacement and/or restoration of teeth by artificial substitutes that are not readily removed from the mouth.

Removable Prosthodontics: The branch of prosthodontics concerned with the replacement of teeth and contiguous structures for edentulous or partially edentulous patients by artificial substitutes that are readily removable from the mouth.

Implant prosthodontics: The phase of prosthodontics concerning the replacement of missing teeth and/or associated structures by restorations that are attached to dental implants.

Maxillofacial prosthetics: The branch of prosthodontics concerned with the restoration and/or replacement of the stomatognathic and craniofacial structures with prostheses that may or may not be removed on a regular or elective basis.

Fixed partial denture: Any dental prosthesis that is luted, screwed or mechanically attached or otherwise securely retained to natural teeth, tooth roots and / or dental implant abutments that furnish the primary support for the dental prosthesis.

INDICATIONS FOR FIXED PARTIAL DENTURE

1. Short edentulous span.
2. Adequate healthy, properly distributed teeth available to serve as abutments.
3. No contraindications are evident.

CONTRAINDICATIONS FOR FIXED PARTIAL DENTURE

1. *Young patients:* Tooth preparation might endanger the pulp.
2. *Advanced age:* Reduced life expectancy and frequently failing general health may limit the long and tedious procedures of FPD.
3. *Increased length of edentulous span:* Adjacent teeth might be over stressed.
4. *Loss of bone in the edentulous area:* FPD does not compensate for loss of bone and soft tissues. An RPD might be a better choice.
5. *Physical or emotional illness of the patient:* Lengthy procedures may turn out to be an ordeal.
6. *Poor general oral health:* FPD requires a highly motivated patient capable of maintaining a good oral hygiene.
7. *Distal edentulous area:* Lack of abutments.
8. *Stabilization of teeth* against anteroposterior and lateral forces: Better established by an RPD.
9. *Severe generalized periodontal disease:* Poor support for FPD and risk of early loss of abutments.
10. *Replacement immediately after extraction:* Alteration in the bone and soft tissue morphology is expected.
11. *Presence of other edentulous areas* in the mouth those are not suitable for FPD: Include this space also in the RPD.

2

Diagnosis and Treatment Planning

Diagnosis: The determination of the nature of a disease[1].

Treatment plan: The sequence of procedures planned for the treatment of a patient after diagnosis.[1]

A thorough diagnosis in the first step in any treatment procedure. Well-thought and well-constructed FPDs may fail because of a wrong diagnosis.[2] To be an accurate diagnostician, the dentist must have a thorough knowledge of both health and disease.[3] Based on the diagnosis, a prognosis is determined and a treatment planned in a stepwise manner. Data may be obtained from medical and dental histories, extra-oral and intraoral examination including examination of pulpal and periodontal health of individual teeth, radiographic and other investigations, articulated diagnostic casts and a survey analysis.

I. PATIENT HISTORY

Personal details of the patient are an integral part of the history to establish an acquaintance with the patient and for future references.

A. Medical History

A series of well-chosen questions is used to elicit a relevant and detailed medical history. Some diseases not only contribute to existing dental disease, but also affect the prognosis of dental treatment. Some conditions may alter the treatment plan. For example,

1. A history of rheumatic heart disease or congenital heart disease may necessitate antibiotic prophylaxis.
2. The presence of pacemaker contraindicates electrosurgical tissue dilation for impression procedures.
3. Use of anticoagulant drugs or hemorrhagic disorders may cause prolonged bleeding and medical treatment is necessary to restore normal coagulating mechanism.
4. History of diabetes mellitus requires careful handling tissues.
5. In hypertensive patients steps should be taken to minimize apprehension to reduce the possibility of cardiovascular accidents.

6. Certain drugs produce chronic xerostomia and facilitate development of cervical dental caries and perodontitis leading to failure of fixed restorations.
7. A history of allergy to drugs also should be noted and used while prescribing drugs to the patient.
8. Local anesthetics are commonly used and any history pertaining to its previous use should be noted.
9. A history of allergy to nickel containing alloys necessitates use of alloys without nickel.
10. Suspected or confirmed carriers of Hepatitis B or AIDS virus require extra precautions to minimize risk to the dentist and auxiliary personnel.
11. Severe eroded teeth may actually be a manifestation of systemic diseases like hiatal hernia, bulimia or anorexia nervosa where regurgitated stomach acids form the etiology.[4]

B. Dental History

Patients past dental experiences, including prior dental treatment should be recorded. Causes for loss of teeth and any complications there on are recorded. The patient's understanding of and attitude toward good oral hygiene practice are important for the success of any fixed prosthesis. The patient should be able to maintain a healthy oral environment before fixed therapy is initiated.

II. CLINICAL EXAMINATION

A. Head and Neck Examination

Size, shape and symmetry of the region along with profile should be recorded. Variations in color, texture, pigmentation, eruptions, cutaneous ulcerations, scars, etc. should be investigated for possible local or systemic diseases. Lymph node enlargements may suggest acute or chronic infections of regional or systemic origin or sometimes neoplasm. A thorough examination of the TMJ and muscles of mastication should be an integral part of the examination procedures. The movements should be smooth and any eccentricities should be investigated.

B. Oral Examination

1. *Lip examination:* The lips should be examined for any signs of malignant neoplastic disease or precancerous lesions. Any suspected lesions should be biopsied for definitive diagnosis. The contour and height of the lips are critical for proper esthetics.
2. *Buccal mucosa* may be a site for leukoplakia, lichen planus, etc. and should be examined thoroughly. Areas of chronic irritation should be examined periodically.

3. *Gingiva:* Many systemic diseases like anemia, leukemia, polycythemia and Addison's disease have a manifestation in the gingiva. The determination of attached and unattached gingiva of the edentulous ridge is of extreme importance in determining placement of pontics.
4. *Tongue:* Usually lesions are traumatic. However, common systemic conditions shown in the tongue are carcinoma, tuberculosis, syphilis, pernicious anemia, herpes and glossitis of vitamin deficiencies. The size and position of the tongue are important in tooth alignment and phonetics.
5. *Palate:* May show changes due to trauma, herpes, necrotizing ulcerative gingivitis, hyperkeratosis following tuberculosis or syphilis, also changes due to smoking.
6. *Floor of the mouth:* Cystic lesions are common. Differentiation from malignant disease is important.
7. *General oral assessment:* Oral hygiene status should be evaluated. Poor oral hygiene can contribute to caries and periodontal breakdown after prosthodontic care. The cause of high caries activity, when present, should be identified and rectified before the commencement of treatment.
8. *Examination of teeth:* Dental prophylaxis is necessary before a thorough examination of teeth is possible. Teeth should be examined for carious lesions, exposed or sensitive root surfaces and wasting diseases—attrition, abrasion or erosion. Restorations should be examined for defective margins or recurrent caries. A detailed periodontal check up involves gingival examination, examination for periodontal pockets, tooth mobility, open contacts, furcation involvement, mucogingival defects and presence of inflammation.
9. *Saliva:* The type and amount of saliva should be noted. Impression making is easier in the presence of serous saliva rather than mucin type. Generally serous saliva is associated with a low caries index.

C. Examination of Occlusion

The examination is to determine if the occlusion of the patient is within normal limits so that the restoration can be designed to maintain the same relationship. When dysfunctional, a decision has to be made to improve the occlusion error before the restoration is initiated or whether the restoration itself can be used to correct the occlusal problems.

- The general alignment of teeth is recorded with a note on features like crowding of teeth, rotations, supra eruption, spacing, type of malocclusion (Angle's) and overlap of teeth. The alteration in alignment of teeth like tipping and crowding necessitate changes in preparation design. Some endodontic and minor orthodontic treatments may be necessary before a final layout of treatment is planned.

- The initial tooth contact (centric relation/terminal hinge position) is recorded and any slide to maximum intercuspation is noted. These features may be evaluated in the presence of other associated problems like increased muscle tone or wear facets.
- Eccentric tooth contacts should be determined and marked. When undesirable, a correction should be made before initiation of treatment.

D. Vitality Testing

Vitality of the teeth especially those that are involved in the design is important. Heat or electric pulp testing may be carried out. If the teeth are found non-vital, their restorability is a concern. A non-restorable tooth is removed and the design of the prosthesis modified (Fig. 2.1).

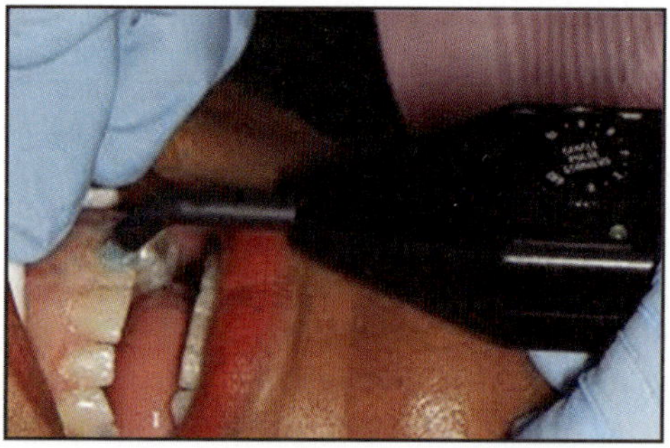

Fig. 2.1: Electric pulp testing

E. TMJ Examination

A detailed examination of the TMJ is essential. The movements should not be restricted. Average mouth opening is greater than 50 mm and any opening less than 35 mm is considered restricted.[5] Any clicking, crepitation or limited movements denote a diseased joint and should be treated before the initiation of treatment, i.e. FPD. Along with the TMJ, the muscles of mastication are also palpated. Any tenderness or spasms require a more detailed examination and treatment.

III. RADIOGRAPHIC EXAMINATION

A minimum of 14 periapical films and 4 bite wing radiographs are made for all FPD patients (Fig. 2.2). Lateral jaw, cephalometric, panoramic or TMJ radiographs are suggested for use when indicated. A variety of information is discernible by a radiographic survey, like:

1. Location and depth of carious lesions.
2. Alveolar bone support around the roots.
3. Presence of bone disease.

4. Width of the periodontal ligament space.
5. Position and height of pulp horns.
6. Osseous resorption and furcation involvements.
7. Length and size of the roots.
8. Crown–root ratio.
9. Axial inclination of teeth (non-parallelism of abutments).
10. Continuity of lamina dura.
11. Previous endodontic restorations—periapical seal and any residual lesions.
12. Presence of periapical disease, root resorption and root fractures.
13. Response of bone to additional stress areas.
14. Retained or impacted teeth.
15. Previous restorations and integrity.
16. Calculus deposits.
17. Evaluation of bone density.

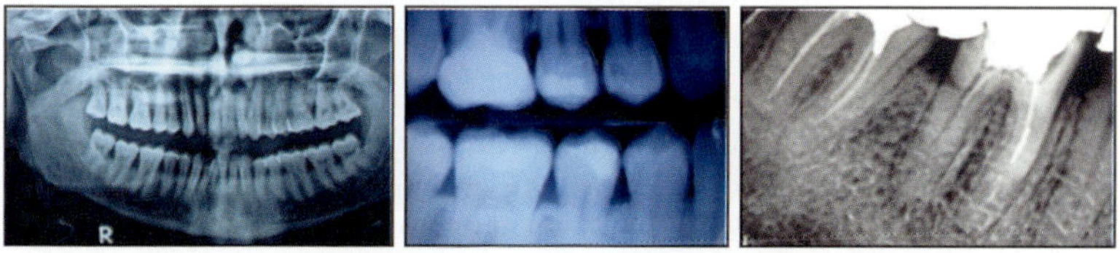

(a) (b) (c)

Fig. 2.2: (a) OPG, (b) Bite wing radiograph, (c) Periapical radiograph

IV. DIAGNOSTIC CASTS

Two weeks after the dental prophylaxis, i.e. after adequate time is given for gingival healing, impressions are made using irreversible hydrocolloid material. The impressions should reproduce all the teeth and associated soft tissue contours. The diagnostic casts not only give information useful in diagnosis but also may be used for fabrication of custom trays for later use.

The various diagnostic information that a diagnostic cast would supply are:

1. Visualization of all edentulous space and their length.
2. Curvature of the arch in the edentulous region.
3. Inclination of all teeth, more importantly the abutment teeth.
4. Occluso-gingival dimension of abutment teeth.
5. Tipping, drifting or rotation of teeth.
6. Spacing between teeth.
7. Number, size and location of wear facets.
8. Occlusal plane discrepancies.
9. Size of pontics needed during diagnostic wax up.
10. Fabrication of provisional restoration.

11. *Occlusal discrepancies:* The diagnostic casts are mounted on a semi-adjustable articulator using a face bow transfer and interocclusal records to simulate jaw movements. Any centric prematurities and excursive interferences are more clearly visible and might require correction before initiation of treatment.

Based on all the data collected, a diagnosis is given. The data is presented for analysis which is then used for a treatment plan formulation. This treatment plan is based on the patients dental needs, mitigated to a variable degree by his or her medical, psychological and personal circumstances and clinical/ dental condition. The treatment plans should be suggested and discussed with the patient with advantages and disadvantages of each.

The treatment mainly follows these steps

1. Education of the patient
2. To establish a disease free environment
3. Assess patients ability to maintain the condition
4. Treatment to improve function and appearance
5. Preventing future disease or maintenance and follow up.

- Education of the patient should be the first step in any treatment plan. The advantages and disadvantages of all treatment options available are discussed. The treatment should begin with the end in mind. A diagnostic wax up may help in visualizing the end product.
- *Disease free environment:*
  - Acute conditions are treated first.
  - Establishing a disease free environment requires assistance from other specialties, discussed in more detail later (Chapter on Periodontal Considerations).
  - Dental caries should be treated and restored. The teeth may be used as abutments at a later stage. Any endodontic treatments should be completed and foundation restorations placed.
  - Teeth with hopeless prognoses should be extracted.
  - The existing periodontal disease is treated in a conventional manner. The etiology for the disease is identified and removed.
  - Minor orthodontic movements may help in achieving better inclination of abutment or space for pontic, etc.
- After the initial therapy is finished, the patient's ability to maintain the health of tissues is assessed before definitive therapy is initiated. A lapse in maintenance may require a repeat of the oral hygiene measures.
- *Definitive therapy:* The scope of fixed prosthodontic treatment ranges from single tooth restorations to full mouth rehabilitation. The fixed prosthodontic treatment may be combined with removable prosthodontics in some instances. The steps in this stage are:

1. Choice of removable or fixed prosthesis. (Refer to indications and contraindications of FPD)
2. Choosing the type of fixed partial denture:
   (a) Fixed-fixed or stationary FPD: Fixed at both ends
   (b) Broken stress FPD: Refer to indications of non-rigid connectors
   (c) Cantilever FPD. Discussed elaborately later
3. Occlusal adjustment—when necessary
4. Selection of abutments
5. Selecting the type of retainer
6. Selecting the type of pontic
7. Designing of components—based on functional and esthetic requirements:
   (a) Pontics (b) Retainers (c) Connectors
8. Tooth preparation
9. Gingival retraction and impression making
10. Temporization
11. Try-in (metal/metal ceramic restorations)
12. Provisional cementation
13. Definitive cementation

When patients require a combination of fixed and removable prosthodontic treatments, removable prosthodontics is usually the last phase. Any preparations thereof should be made priorly in the castings, e.g. rest seat preparations, ledges for reciprocal arm, undercut for the retainer arm, etc. Once the castings are cemented, further procedures for construction of the RPD are carried out.

- *Maintenance and follow-up:* Any treatment regime is incomplete without proper maintenance and follow-up. The patient is inspected at regular intervals to determine the health of tissues and adequacy of restoration function and esthetics. Postoperative care is a key for long-term service of the prosthesis and a chapter is dedicated for the same.

REFERENCES

1. Glossary of Prosthodontic Terms. *J. Prosthet. Dent* 2005; 94:10–92.
2. Bull A.W. Diagnosis: A factor in the success of fixed partial dentures. *J. Prosthet. Dent* 1970; 24:498–502.
3. Brehm T.W. Diagnosis and treatment planning for fixed prosthodontics. *J. Prosthet. Dent* 1973; 30:876–81.
4. Milosevic A. Eating disorders and the dentist, *Br. Dent. J* 1999;186:109–13.
5. Pullinger A.G., Liu S., Tay G.D. Differences between sexes in maximum jaw opening when corrected to body size, *J. Oral Rehabil* 1987;14:291–9.

3 Periodontal Considerations in FPD

Periodontia cannot be successfully divorced from any branch of dentistry.[1] A healthy periodontium is critical for the success of an FPD. The assessment of the periodontal status of the involved abutment teeth gives a fair indication of the prognosis of the prosthesis. It is important to achieve a healthy periodontium before the FPD is planned and it should be possible to maintain the status during the service of the prosthesis for a longer life of the prosthesis. The services of a periodontist should be employed whenever required. A team approach in treating the patient is fast replacing the individual approach for effective care.[2]

An adequate knowledge of the normal periodontium is an essential part of the periodontal considerations but a detailed discussion on the same is beyond the scope of this book.

The periodontal considerations in FPD can be discussed under:

I. Periodontal procedures to improve the abutment health/preparation of the periodontium.
II. Study of the effect of FPD on the periodontal status/restoration of periodontium interrelationships.
III. FPD for a periodontally compromised situation.

I. PREPARATION OF PERIODONTIUM FOR RESTORATIVE DENTISTRY

The procedures in this phase include all those steps carried out to bring back the periodontium into a state of complete health. Or, at least to a state where further progression of the disease is stopped. The procedures are divided into two categories:

A. Initial/preliminary procedures
B. Definitive/secondary procedures

A. Initial Procedures

These are the treatments carried out before an evaluation for requirement of surgical treatments is made. It involves simple procedures and is usually the only treatment required in the initial stages of periodontal disease. The aim of these procedures is to obtain and maintain a plaque free environment.

1. Minimize Plaque

Bacterial plaque forms on all surfaces of the teeth and in all mouths. It is formed more in some mouths compared to some others and it is more prevalent in the gingival third of the teeth. The bacteria in the plaque produce toxins that are harmful to the health of the periodontium. Hence continuous removal of plaque is mandatory for the health of the tissues.

a. *Patient education:* The patient needs to be educated regarding the methods of plaque removal which include tooth brushing, flossing and use of other oral hygiene aids. Tooth brushing is a very effective method of plaque removal based on the type of brush used, technique employed and frequency of brushing. The bass sulcular method of brushing is the most preferred as it effectively cleans the sulci where the margins of the restorations are placed (Fig. 3.1).

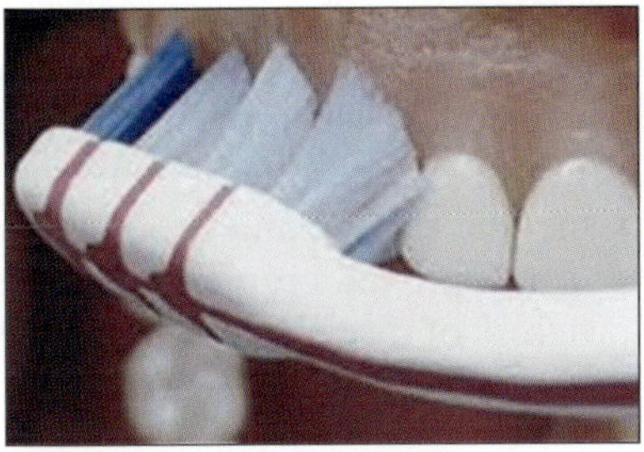

Fig. 3.1: Brushing

The dental floss cleans the inter-proximal areas of teeth. The patient is educated on the effective use of floss. Just brushing and no flossing usually leave 40% of the tooth surfaces unclean. Use of other aids like tooth picks, interdental stimulators, inter-proximal brushes or electric tooth brushes are beneficial in some circumstances and the patient should be educated about the same. Disclosing agents help to visualize areas where plaque control is difficult or deficient. A well-educated and motivated patient goes a long way in the success of an FPD.

b. *Scaling and polishing:* Removal of calculus and polishing the coronal portion of the tooth are the first steps in debridement of the teeth. Supragingival scaling is done first followed by a time interval. The gingiva responds to this treatment by reduction in inflammation, bleeding and size. The subgingival calculus becomes visible and is then removed. Polishing removes the scratches made during scaling in turn reducing plaque accumulation (Fig. 3.2).

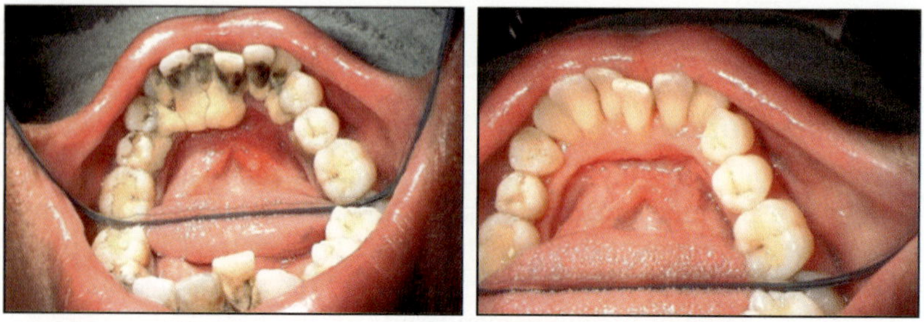

Before After

Fig. 3.2: Supragingival and subgingival deposits

A sub-clinical level of inflammation is always present and scaling and polishing should be a mandatory procedure. The gingival level is important as it is an important consideration in the placement of finish lines.

c. *Root planing:* Root planing is the process by which residual embedded calculus and portions of cementum are removed from the roots to produce a smooth, hard, clean surface. The root surface/cementum is irregular and usually microorganisms and endotoxins get embedded into them. Thus, removal of a portion of cementum is necessary. The curettage of soft issue that accompanies root planing removes a layer of inflamed tissue. An improved oral hygiene practice by the patient usually halts the progress of disease and further treatment may not be necessary.

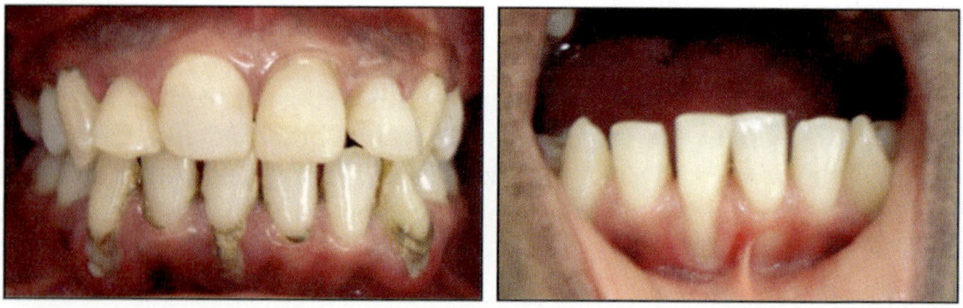

Before After

Fig. 3.3: Supragingival and subgingival deposits

2. Correction of Defective Restorations

Overhanging margins, improper proximal contours/ encroachment of gingival embrasures, open contacts that form areas of food impaction—all these require correction before the restoration is initiated. These, if left untreated, may cause widespread periodontal involvement, finally leading to the failure of an FPD.

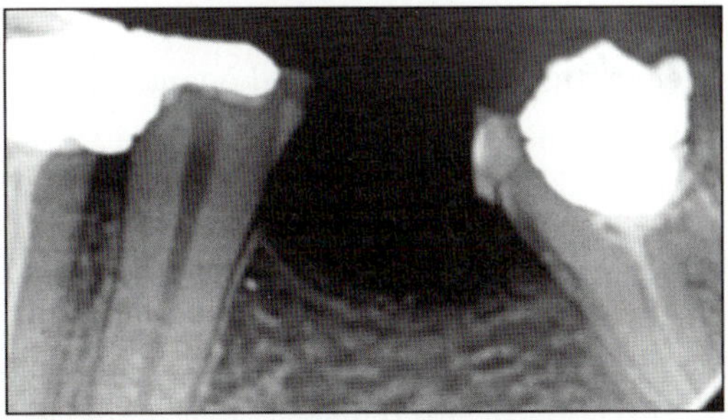

Fig. 3.4

3. Splinting

Teeth become mobile when subjected to heavy occlusal forces, especially when the bone support is compromised. These teeth require a corrective treatment when they cause discomfort to the patient or when the mobility is progressive. The treatment include correction of occlusal forces acting on the teeth and splinting, i.e. joining together of two or more teeth for stabilization.

If the destructive forces are modified and teeth splinted, mobile teeth become firm. However, if the teeth are splinted without modification of forces, the entire splint can become unstable.[2] Splinting may be accomplished by provisional restorations, bonding or partial coverage metal restorations.

4. Planned Tooth Removal

Teeth that are hopelessly involved periodontally and those that are non-restorable should be extracted during initial therapeutic procedures. Early extraction allows the socket areas to heal and also provides better access for plaque control of adjacent tooth surfaces. The space created and opposing occlusion can be maintained by fabricating provisional RPD or FPD.

Periodontally weak left incisors are best removed to use other teeth as abutments (Fig. 3.5).

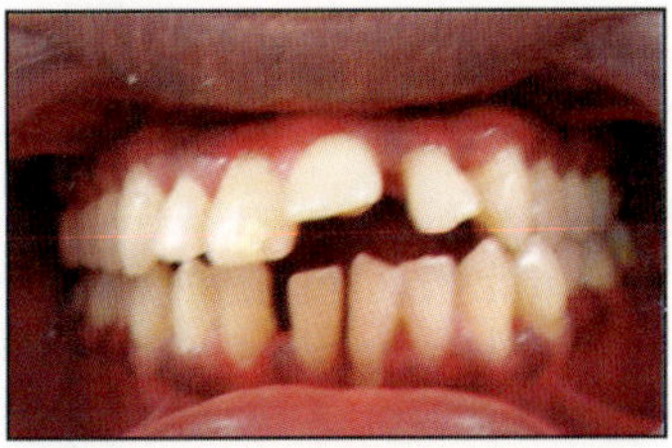

Fig. 3.5: Periodontally weak left incisors are best removed to use other teeth as abutments

5. Adjunctive Orthodontic Therapy

There are several benefits of adjunctive orthodontic therapy that include:

i. Improved alignment of malposed or crowded teeth permits better access to all surfaces of the teeth.
ii. Vertical tooth repositioning may sometime eliminate the need for resective osseous surgery. For example, correction of hemiseptal defects.
iii. Orthodontic treatment may help improve the esthetics of maxillary gingiva by correction of discrepancies that might otherwise require recontouring with or without bone removal.
iv. When a tooth/root fractures close to the socket margin, it might leave insufficient coronal structure to support a restoration. The root may be orthodontically extruded to give sufficient resistance and retention form for the final restoration.
v. Orthodontic separation may be used to reduce root proximities. The roots may or may not require further treatment.
vi. Orthodontic treatment can be used to improve adjacent tooth positions before implant placements.

B. Definitive Procedures

A diligent effort during initial therapy cuts the progress of disease. When damage caused by the disease is minimal, no further treatment may be necessary. The restorative treatment is initiated when the patient shows competence in the maintenance of a disease/plaque free environment.

However, when the damages of the disease have been profound, like substantial root exposures, persistent probing depths, hypertrophy of gingiva, or loss of bone, the more definitive or surgical procedures are required. These procedures also contribute for improving the prognosis of the FPD.

Surgical Therapy

A detailed description of all periodontal surgeries may be found in the relevant textbooks of periodontics. A short discussion of the various surgical procedures is given here.

A. Soft tissue procedures

1. *Gingivectomy*: Gingivectomy means the excision of gingiva. It removes the pocket wall and provides visibility and accessibility for complete calculus removal and smoothening of roots. Resection is confined to keratinized gingiva (Fig. 3.6).

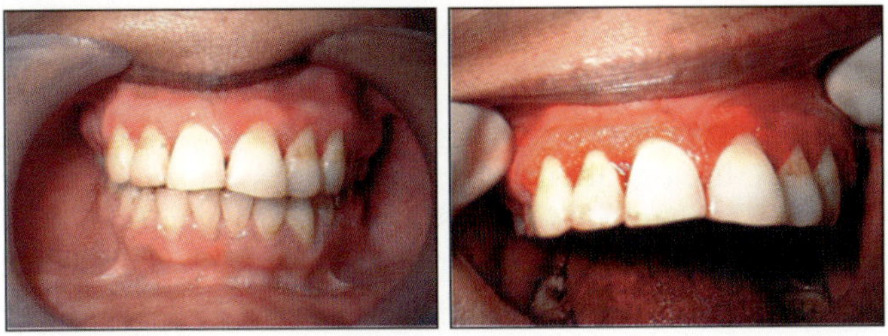

Fig. 3.6: Gingivectomy in the upper anterior quadrant

Indications

1. Elimination of supra-bony pocket, if the pocket wall is fibrous and firm
2. Elimination of gingival enlargements, e.g. those following hydantoin therapy
3. Elimination of supra-bony periodontal abscesses.

Contraindications

1. Absence of attached keratinized tissue
2. The need for bone surgery or examination of bone shape and morphology
3. If it leaves the root exposed specially in the esthetic regions.

2. *Open debridement:* A periodontal flap, usually a modified Wildman flap, is opened to gain access to the root surfaces. The area is debrided and the flap is closed in intimate adaptation to the tooth (Fig. 3.7).

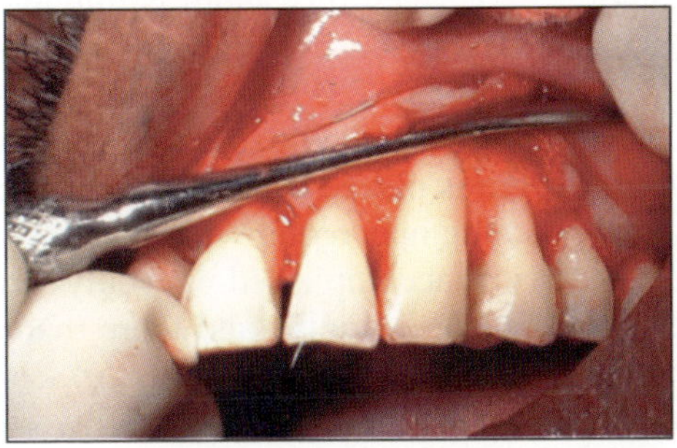

Fig. 3.7: Flap opened for debridement of the area

3. *Management of mucogingival problems:* The most common reason why a periodontal surgery for mucosal repair is required is to increase the widths of keratinized gingiva and to achieve root coverage. Various surgical procedures that are carried out include—free autogenous gingival graft, laterally or coronally positioned pedicle graft and sub-

epithelial connective tissue graft. A detailed discussion of the techniques may be found in the periodontal textbooks.

B. Hard-tissue procedures

The periodontal disease, after the active phase is waded off, might have left certain bone topography of areas where plaque control is difficult or even impossible. The common occurrences are:

1. Irregular pattern of bone loss leading to intrabony pockets.
2. Exposed root furcations.

While treating these conditions, a decision needs to be made about the mode of treatment, i.e. either by induction of new bone formation with resulting new attachment or by removal and reshaping of bone in the area to facilitate easy plaque removal and stop progress of disease (resective or reconstructive periodontal surgeries).

C. Crown-lengthening procedures

Indications

1. Improve appearance of an anterior tooth
2. Clinical crown too short to provide adequate retention and resistance form
3. To adjust gingival levels for aesthetics
4. Subgingival caries or fracture.

It is important that crown-lengthening procedures should not impinge on the biologic width. The biologic width is defined as the physiologic dimension of the functional epithelium and connective tissue attachment and is approximately 2 mm, when this width is impinged upon, it may result in gingival inflammation, pocket formation and alveolar bone loss.

It is recommended that at least 3.0 mm distance exists between bone crest and gingival margin. This would not breach the biologic width even when the restoration margin is placed 0.5 mm into the gingival sulcus.

Surgical crown-lengthening may require removal of both hard and soft tissues. The procedure can be accomplished with only soft tissue removal when there is adequate attached gingiva and more than 3 mm of tissue coronal to bone crest. When less than 3 mm of soft tissue is present, a recontouring of alveolar bone is required before soft tissue correction can be made (Fig. 3.8).

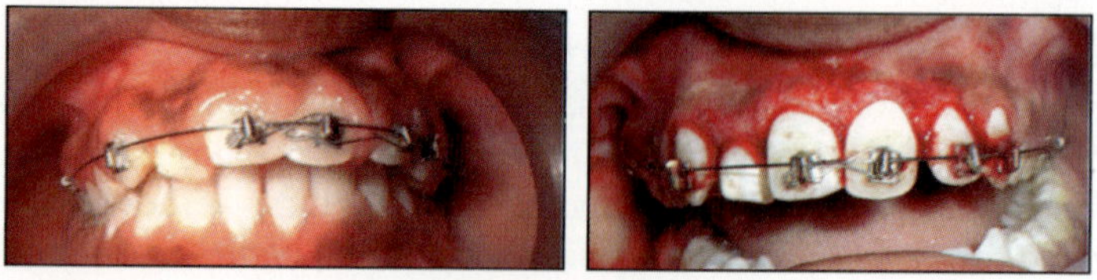

Fig. 3.8: Surgical crown-lengthening

Crown-lengthening may also be accomplished with combined orthodontic periodontal techniques. Sometimes it is better to expose the subgingival fracture or caries with extrusion and restore the tooth with margins on sound tooth structure.

The goals to be achieved with this phase of the treatment are thus:

1. Ensure stable gingival margins before tooth preparation. Healthy tissues tend to change less as a result of subgingival restorative treatment, and are also less likely to bleed.
2. Provide adequate tooth length for retention, access for tooth preparation, impression making and finishing of restorative margins.
3. Reduce traumatic forces on the tooth thus reducing tooth mobility, discomfort and possibly the rate of attachment loss.

II. RESTORATION OF PERIODONTIUM INTERRELATIONSHIPS

The restoration should be built in harmony with the surrounding periodontal issues, so that they remain healthy and in turn restorations survive for a long term. The restoration should function in the mouth without injuring the adjacent tissues while fulfilling the esthetic requirements. The features of the restoration that should be closely monitored for periodontal health are individually discussed.

1. Margin Placement and Biologic Width

The various locations for margin placement have included:

i. The base of the gingival crevice[3]
ii. Half the distance between the base of gingival crevice and the gingival margin[4]
iii. Slightly below the gingival margin[5]
iv. At the crest of the gingival margin[6]
v. Supragingivally.[7,8]

G.V. Black advocated subgingival margins as he considered this a "caries-free zone." Orban and other researchers later found that the clean area on extracted teeth were nothing but the location of the epithelial attachment. Orban, as early as 1940, proposed supragingival margins.[9]

Plaque accumulation, inflammation and gingivitis occur more frequently in teeth with subgingival margins.[6,7] The supragingival margin will have the least impact on the periodontium. With the advent of the recent translucent restorative materials, adhesive dentistry and resin cements, the surpragingival margins may be placed even in esthetic areas and should be chosen whenever possible. The only logical indications for subgingival margins are:

1. Esthetic demands
2. Caries removal

3. Subgingival tooth fracture
4. To cover existing subgingival restoration
5. To gain needed crown length
6. To provide a more favorable crown contour
7. An existing full coverage restoration with subgingival margins

Biologic width also has an important role in preserving healthy gingival tissues. It is the dimension of space that the healthy gingival tissues occupy above the alveolar bone. Clinically, when the restoration margin is placed 2 mm or less away from the alveolar bone, it is diagnosed as a biologic width violation. This may lead to either bone loss along with gingival tissue recession or bone level renaming unchanged but gingival inflammation develops and persists. The type of reaction seen depends on the type of gingiva and the amount of scalloping in the periodontium. It has been found that highly scalloped, thin gingiva is more prone to recession than a flat periodontium with thick fibrous tissue.

The violation of biologic width should be the remedied as early as possible. This is done either by surgery to alter the bone level or by moving the restoration margin away from the bone by orthodontic extrusion (Fig. 3.9).

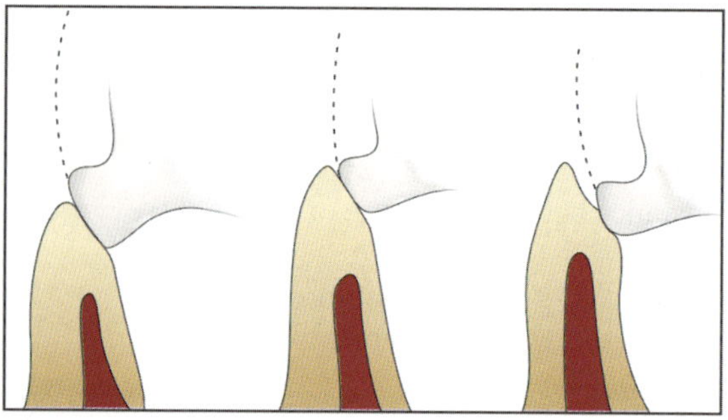

Fig. 3.9: Supragingival, equigingival and subgingival location of finish line

2. Crown Contours

Contours of the crown are extremely important for maintenance of periodontal health. The evolution of ideal contours has progressed through different stages or theories. The prominent of them being

a. Gingival protection theory[10,11]
b. Muscle action theory[12,13]
c. Access for oral hygiene[14]

The gingival protection theory advocated the use of overcontoured restorations so as to deflect the masticated food away from the gingival margin and sulcus, thus protecting the gingiva (Fig. 3.10). However, when a cause and effect relationship was found between plaque, gingivitis and interrelationship of food impaction, the periodontal disease appeared slight.[14,15] This indicates that plaque accumulation is a bigger factor in periodontal disease than food impaction.

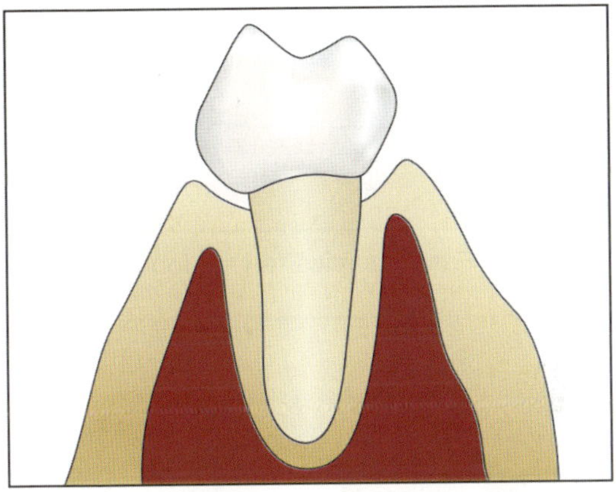

Fig. 3.10: Overcontoured restorations to deflect food away from gingiva

The muscle action theory claimed that the normal action of musculature has a cleaning action on the gingiva. However, these self-cleansing mechanisms have been shown to be ineffective in the absence of oral hygiene measures.[14,16]

Theory of access for oral hygiene is based on the concept that plaque is the prime etiologic factor in caries and gingivitis. They advocated the use of crown contours that facilitate plaque removal, not hinder it. The concept used flat buccal and lingual contours along with open embrasures for easy cleansing. Under contouring it does not produce any adverse effect on the periodontium. When esthetics permit, flatter contours are preferable to fat contours.

3. Pontic Design

The pontic should be designed to have minimal tissue contact and adequate accessibility for oral hygiene. The open embrasures adjacent to abutments allow room for inter-proximal tissue health and access for oral hygiene. The finish of the undersurface of pontic is more important than the material itself. The occlusal surface should not be narrowed arbitrarily as this may create a food impaction and/or plaque retention situation similar to a malposed tooth. The embrasure space between two adjacent pontics is usually closed. This provides additional strength to the restoration, reduces food and plaque retention, also facilitates oral hygiene procedures under pontic areas (Figs. 3.11 and 3.12).[17]

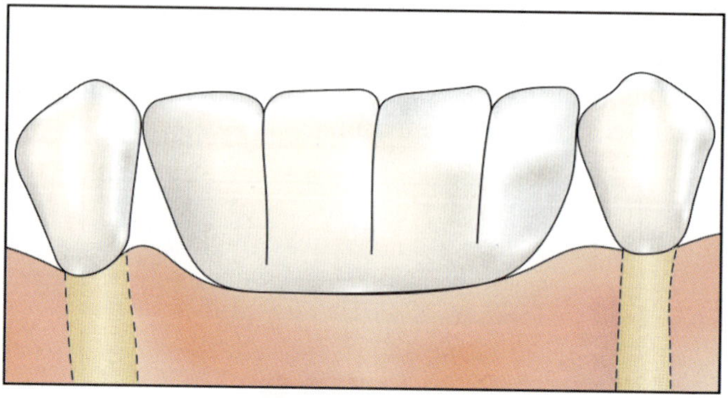

Fig. 3.11: Fused pontics reduce food impaction

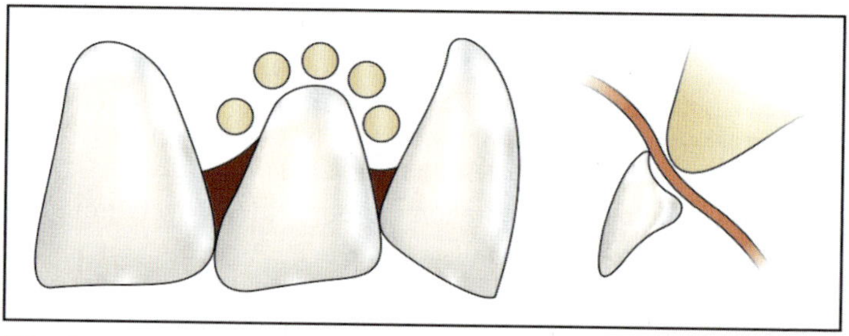

Fig. 3.12: Dental floss used to clean the undersurface of pontics

4. Provisional Restorations

The three critical areas that must be effectively managed to produce a favorable biologic response to provisional restorations are marginal fit, crown contours and surface finish. All of these should be appropriate so as to maintain the health and position of gingival tissues until final restorations are delivered.

Short temporary crown margins allow migration of gingiva over the finish line. This eventually prevents seating of final crown leaving a cement space, which may dissolve and leave an open margin. Overcontoured restorations cause gingival recession, the chances being higher with longer span of use. These unfavorable changes in tissue architecture can compromise the success of the final restoration.

5. Marginal Fit

The fit of margins is an extremely important consideration. Open margins harbor a large number of bacteria that are responsible for causing inflammation in gingiva. Open margins may lead to sensitive restoration following loss of cement. They may even be starting points for carious lesions (Fig. 3.13).

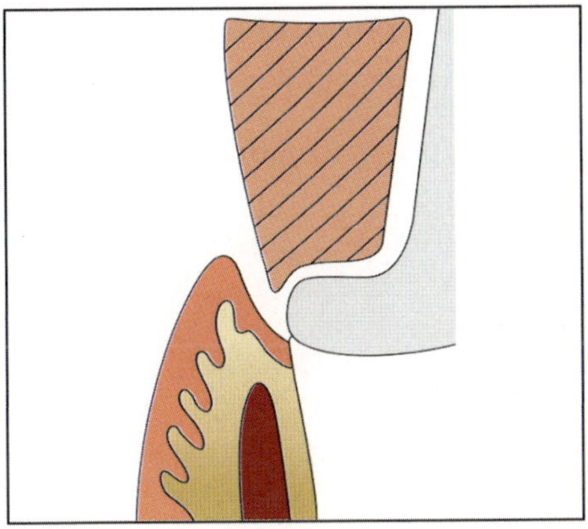

Fig. 3.13: Close adaptation of margins is important for gingival health

6. Full Coverage vs Partial Coverage

Partial coverage restorations have better periodontal response because of less gingival involvement. The margins are usually supragingival with better access for hygiene.

7. Gingival Retraction and Impression Making

- Soft tissue trauma is a common occurrence when excessive pressure is applied in mechanical gingival retraction. The gingiva may heal with slight recession exposing the margins of the final restoration.
- The cord should be gently pushed into the gingival sulcus with specially designed bladed instruments or a blunted periodontal probe.
- When a double cord technique is used, the thinner cord is placed deeper to suit the shape of the sulcus.
- The thickness of cord selected should be according to the type of gingiva. For example, thin firmly adapted tissue requires smallest cord, whereas a medium size cord is indicated when greater tissue bulk is encountered.
- Electrosurgical tissue displacement should be done only in the presence of healthy periodontal tissue, otherwise significant changes in gingival form or height may occur on healing.
- On removal of the impression, both the sulcus and the impression should be thoroughly observed for any tears leaving some material in the sulcus. Any unnoticed remains of the impression material may initiate an inflammatory process in the periodontium.

8. Location of Contact Areas

- The contact area should be in the occlusal or incisal third.
- Large contact areas create a large col that is sensitive to plaque. Hence contact areas should be small.[18]

- In the anterior region, the contact is placed slightly lingual to develop esthetic contours in the restoration.
- It is recommended to place contact areas as far occlusally as possible to facilitate interproximal plaque control (Fig. 3.14).[19]

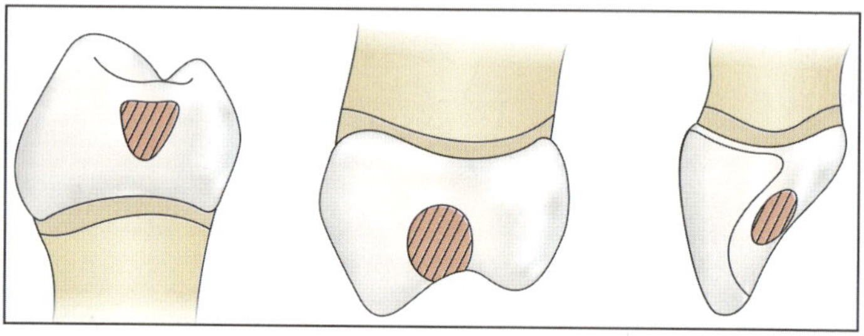

Fig. 3.14: Location of contact areas for gingival health and esthetics

III. PERIODONTALLY WEAKENED TEETH

With advanced periodontal treatment techniques, even the severely involved teeth can be saved. However, they retain some residual features of the disease like exposed roots, furcations or altered crown root ratio. Although such teeth are not the most ideal abutments, they are still viable and can be used satisfactorily. These require certain modification of the preparation or the tooth itself before they are a safe risk as abutments. What such treatment produces are discussed here.

1. Loss of Gingival Height

The preparation of the abutment will require certain modifications. The ideal location of the finish line, i.e. on the enamel away from the gingival sulcus is no longer possible. The preparation is usually extended to cover the exposed root surface.

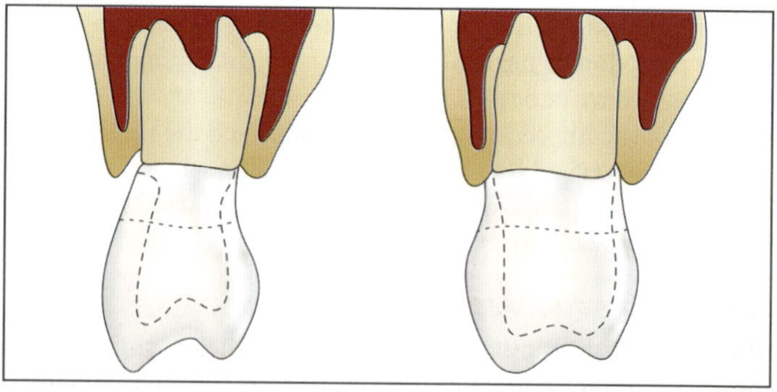

Fig. 3.15: Maxillary premolar prepared with shoulder and chamfer finish lines

A shoulder finish line is a poor choice. The root usually has a smaller diameter than the crown and the axial reduction may be very close to the pulp to endanger tooth vitality. This amount of preparation also weakens the tooth. Also the shoulder may concentrate stresses that could fracture the tooth. A chamfer finish line will result in approximately the same depth of axial reduction at the apical position as the shoulder would at its usual level.

The type of contour provided to the restoration in the gingival half will depend on the topography and type of gingiva present.

2. Root Exposure Extending Close to Furcation

The furcation is the area where the root trunk divides into two or three roots. There are usually vertical concavities or flutes extending from the actual furcation towards the cemento-enamel junction on the root trunk. This causes a change in the design of tooth preparation as well as the restoration/crown.

The axial surfaces of the tooth preparation occlusal to the inversion of the gingival finish line must also exhibit vertical concavities or flutes. The axial contours of crowns placed on teeth with finish lines extending to these flutes must also reflect the concavity rising from the furcation flute. The crown should follow the curvature of the flute in the area and not the original crown contours to ensure adequate plaque control.[20] If these contours are not followed, it creates a horizontal ridge in the gingival 1/3rd that acts as a plaque retaining area.

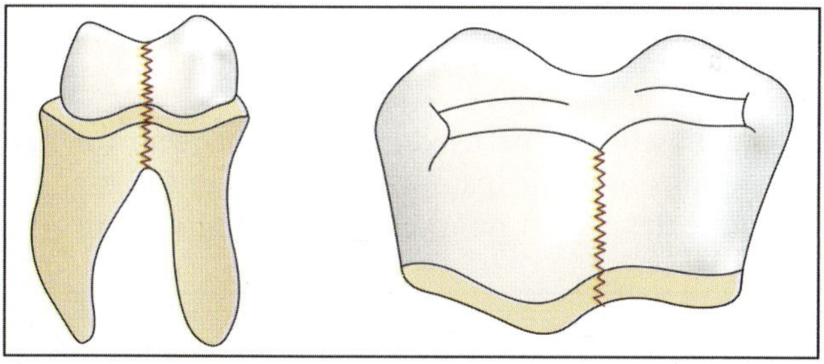

Fig. 3.16: Flutes from furcation is replicated in the crown

3. Compromised Periodontal Support of One Root in a Multirooted Tooth

The periodontal support of the roots is a key factor in the decision to use a tooth as an abutment. When one root of the tooth has compromised support, the tooth can still be salvaged by removal of the root with or without the removal of a part of the crown. Such a treatment is called *radectomy* or *root resection*. A hemisection is a procedure in which the tooth is separated through the crown and the furcation, producing two essentially equal-sized tooth.

Root Resection or Root Amputation

Indications[21]

1. Severe loss of bone or attachment around one root.
2. To eradicate areas of the tooth that create problems in the maintenance of good hygiene and plaque control.
3. To change the furcation anatomy and make it easily cleansable.
4. To salvage teeth with endodontic problems of that root, including perforations, irretrievable broken instruments, anatomy that prevents successful endodontics, etc.
5. Fractured root.
6. When roots of two adjacent teeth are in such close proximity that the embrasure space is obliterated, it improves the prognosis of the adjacent tooth.
7. Resorption—internal or external.
8. Severe caries involving the root.
9. Severe sensitivity of one root.
10. Removal to improve prognosis of the next tooth.

Contraindications[21,22]

1. Fused roots, or closely approximated roots of the same tooth. It does not leave enough interradicular bone to support the remaining root.
2. The furcation is too far apical, e.g. maxillary 1st premolars.
3. When alveolar support has been lost uniformly around all of the roots.
4. When the tooth cannot be successfully treated endodontically.

Advantages

1. The resected teeth can be used as abutment teeth for fixed partial dentures, splints or vertical stops for cantilever FPDs.
2. May preclude the need for a removable partial denture.

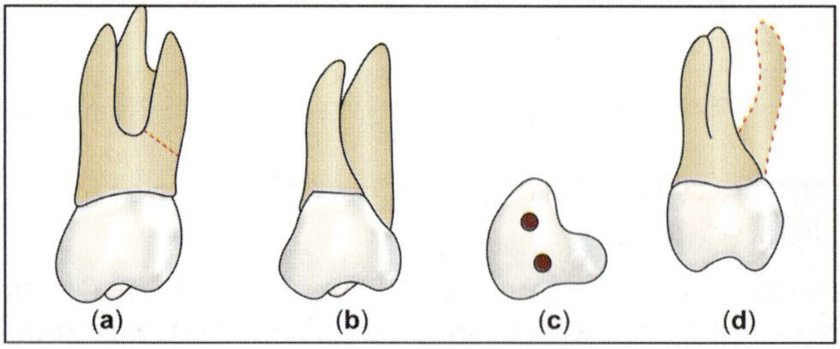

Fig. 3.17: (a) Incision line marked on the distal root of maxillary molar, (b) Root resected and margins smoothened, (c) Cross-sectional view, (d) Palatal view after root amputation

Disadvantages

1. Reduced load bearing ability because of diminished attachment area.
2. Demanding technique.
3. Chances of leaving a ridge that may act as a plaque retaining area.
4. Need for a dowel and core to restore the teeth.
5. Need for endodontic treatment before the tooth can be used as abutment.

Restoration

A cast post and core may be indicated to create an adequate foundation for final restoration. Appropriate contours must be developed in the restoration for access towards hygiene. Facially and lingually, the contours of the crown should be essentially a straight line from the margin coronally. Inter-proximally, the contours are straight in the gingival half and slightly convex coronally as it slopes to the contact point. When the inter-proximal areas of the root trunk exhibit concavities, the gingival embrasure form of the restoration must be fluted into these areas so that the surfaces can be accessed with an inter-proximal brush.

The kind of contour developed in a restoration depends on which roots are amputated (Figs 3.18 to 3.21). Esthetics is usually not a concern unless a maxillary first molar is the involved tooth. When the mesiobuccal root is amputated, it is better to create an artificial mesiobuccal root with a normal crown contour coronal to it and a furcation made of the restorative material that is easily cleanable with an interdental brush.

Clinical presentation

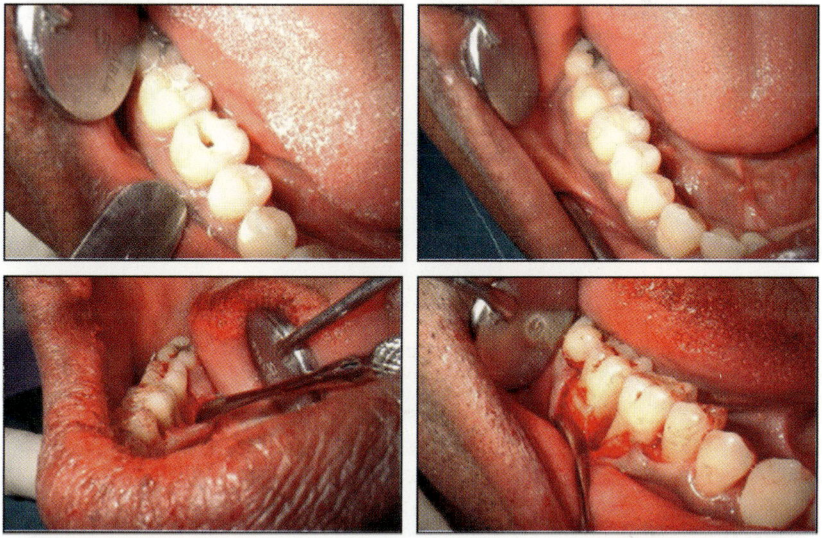

Fig. 3.18: Poor bone support in the distal root of mandibular first molar

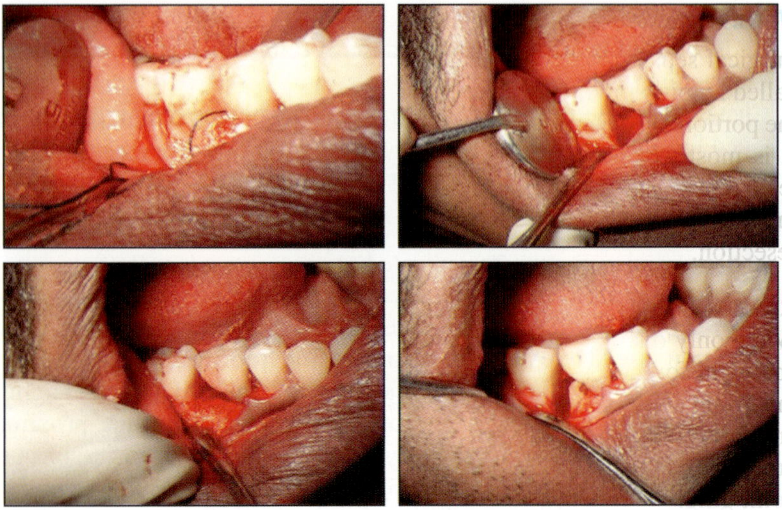

Fig. 3.19: Distal root amputated

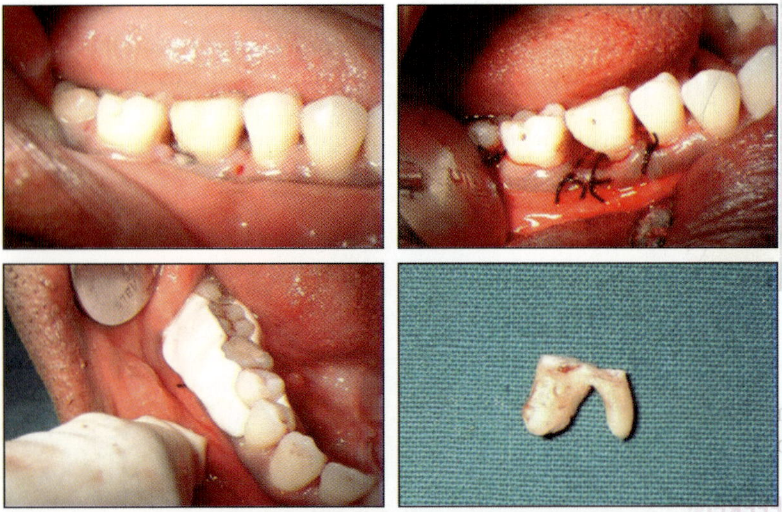

Fig. 3.20: Sutures and healing pack placed

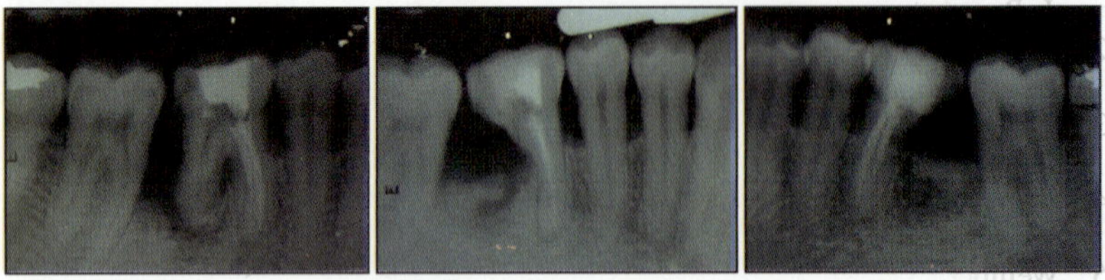

Fig. 3.21: Preoperative and postoperative radiographs

Hemisection

Surgical separation of a multi-rooted tooth through the furcation area is called hemisection. The two sections may be retained as separate units or the portion that has compromised support removed and the other retained. It is most frequently performed on mandibular molars. Since it leaves teeth equal to premolars, the procedure is also called bicuspidization. The indications and contraindications of hemisection are the same as root resection.

Restoration

When only one-half of the tooth is retained, the tooth can be used as an abutment for a short span FPD or RPD. If both roots are maintained, it is important that they be separated from each other to allow normal gingival embrasures. Separation may be accomplished by moving the roots apart orthodontically or designing of crowns such that they taper from the contact point gingivally leaving sufficient embrasure space.

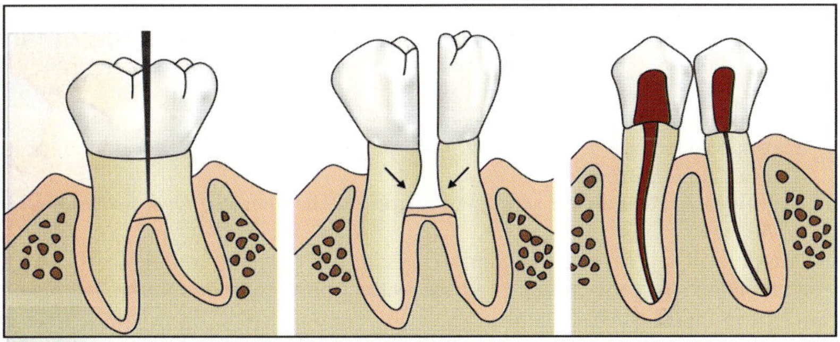

Fig. 3.22: Steps in hemisection of mandibular molar

Joint consultations by the periodontist and prosthodontist will lead to the best possible solutions for treatment with the least confusion and delay to the patient.[23]

REFERENCES

1. Kimball H.D. The role of periodontia in prosthetic dentistry, *J. Prosthet. Dent* 1951; 1:286–94.
2. Krajicek D.D. Periodontal considerations for prosthetic patients, *J. Prosthet. Dent* 1973; 30:15–18.
3. Stein R., Glickman I., Prosthetic considerations essential for gingival health. Dent Clin North Am 1960; 4:177.
4. Tylman S.D. The theory and practice of crown and fixed partial prosthodontics, 6th ed., St Louis: Mosby 1970, p. 94.
5. Weinberg L.A. Esthetics and the gingival in full coverage, *J. Prosthet. Dent* 1960; 10:737–44.

6. Marcum J. The effect of crown marginal depth upon gingival tissue, *J. Prosthet. Dent* 1967; 17:479–87.
7. Silness J. Periodontal conditions in patients treated with dental bridges. Part III. The relationship between the location of crown margin and the periodontal condition, *J. Periodont. Res* 1970; 5:225–9.
8. Eissman H., Radke R., Noble W. Physiologic design criteria for fixed dental restorations. *Dent Clin North Am* 1971; 15:543.
9. Orban B. Biological considerations in restorative dentistry, *J. Am. Dent. Assoc* 1941; 28:1069.
10. Henry P., Johnston J., Mitchell D. Tissue changes beneath fixed partial dentures, *J. Prosthet. Dent* 1966; 16:937–47.
11. Wheeler RC. Complete crown form and the periodontium, *J. Prosthet. Dent* 1961; 11:722–34.
12. Morris M. Artificial crown contours and gingival health, *J. Prosthet. Dent* 1962; 12:1146–56.
13. Wagman S.S. The role of coronal contour in gingival health. *J. Prosthet. Dent* 1977; 37:280–7.
14. Loe H., Theilade E., Jensen S. Experimental gingivitis in man, *J. Periodont.* 1965; 36:177.
15. Schwartz R., Massler M., LeBeau L. Gingival reactions to different types of tooth accumulated materials, *J. Periodont* 1971; 42:144.
16. Lindhe J., Wicen P., the effects on the gingivae of chewing fibrous foods, *J. Periodont. Res* 1969; 4:193–201.
17. Behrend D.A., The mandibular posterior fixed partial denture, *J. Prosthet. Dent* 1977; 37:622–38.
18. Hazen S., Osborne J. Relationship of operative dentistry to periodontal health, *Dent Clin North Am* 1967; 11:245.
19. Ramfjord S. Periodontal aspects of restorative dentistry, *J. Oral Rehabil.* 1974, 1:107.
20. Yuodelis R., Weaver J., Sapkos S. Facial and lingual contours of artificial complete crown restorations and their effect on the periodontium. *J. Prosthet. Dent* 1973; 29:61–6.
21. Baima R.F. Considerations for furcation treatment. II. Periodontal therapy. *J. Prosthet. Dent* 1987; 57:400.
22. Fournier DF. Odontic trisection: An alternative therapy. *J. Prosthet. Dent* 1987; 57:397–400.
23. Nassif J., Blumenfeld W.L., Joint consultation services by the periodontist and prosthodontist, *J. Prosthet. Dent* 1973; 29:55–60.

4

Restoration of Carious and Endodontically Treated Teeth

Bygone are the days when extraction used to be the choice of treatment for teeth with extensive caries or decay. Preservation of teeth is one of the prime objectives of dental practice today. Teeth with cavities but are vital and teeth that have become non-vital are all treated successfully. Endodontic therapy has provided the solution to maintain mutilated teeth and aid them to resume full function. They can serve satisfactorily standing alone or as an abutment for fixed and removable prosthesis.

VITAL TEETH

- Surface lesions that would be entirely removed during tooth preparations do not need any special attention.
- Dental cement may be used to fill small defects or undercut areas in the preparation intraorally.
- All carious lesions are restored to full contour. The teeth and restoration together is then prepared to receive the retainer.
- In extensively damaged vital teeth, some improvement in retention may be obtained by placement of grooves, pinholes and box walls in sound dentin. For these adjuncts to be useful they should be at least 1.5 mm away from the outer surface of the tooth.
- Sometimes, an extensively damaged tooth may have to be devitalized to improve the retention and resistance form of the restoration.

NON-VITAL TEETH

i. *Non-RCT treated tooth:* Every non-vital tooth should be treated endodontically and left in the mouth for a period of time to evaluate its prognosis. The remaining steps are similar to an RCT treated tooth.
ii. *RCT treated tooth:* All RCT treated teeth need to be assessed before any further treatments are planned.

ASSESSMENT OF ENDOTREATED TEETH

Before the restoration of the endodontically treated teeth, it should be assessed for the following factors:[1]

1. Good apical seal—inadequate fillings should be re-treated.
2. No sensitivity to pressure.
3. No exudates.
4. No fistula.
5. No apical sensitivity.
6. No active inflammation.
7. Favorable soft tissue health.
8. Adequate bone support around the roots.

Endodontically treated teeth usually have lost a lot of tooth structure due to caries, previous restorations, fractures or endodontic treatment. Once the endotreatment is complete, the tooth needs to be restored to its full form using various treatment methods. The kind of treatment chosen for such a tooth would depend on

1. The amount of remaining coronal tooth structure
2. The type of tooth (incisor, canine, premolar or molar)
3. The role the tooth has to assume after restoration
   i. Single unit
   ii. Abutment for RPD or overdenture
   iii. Abutment for FPD.

RESTORATIONS

Simple Filling

Indicated when the coronal structure is largely intact.

a. *Silver amalgam or miracle mix:* Class I access cavity fillings in posterior teeth with intact marginal ridges and areas not subjected to excessive occlusal forces.
b. *GIC restorations:* Simple access cavity fillings in the anterior teeth involving only the palatal surface and without discoloration.
c. *Composite resin restorations:* Otherwise intact anterior teeth with minimal proximal carious lesions.

Full Coverage Restorations

Anterior and posterior teeth might need full coverage restorations or crowns. The access cavity is filled and the tooth restored to its full form before it is prepared for receiving a crown. Such a procedure is called core buildup. The need for such restorations may be decided by:

a. Significant loss of tooth structure, b. discoloration or other esthetic requirements. Discoloration may sometimes be effectively treated with bleaching,[2] c. restoration of occlusion. d. areas of mouth with a high risk of fracture, e. the tooth is to act as an abutment for RPD or FPD. They are more than four times as likely to fail as compared to them not serving as abutments.[3]

The various full coverage restorations are metal, metal-ceramic or all ceramic crowns. Based on the clinical situation and patient desires, an appropriate choice of restoration is made.

Post and Core Restorations

History

The advent of post and core first began in 18th century when wooden wedges were inserted into root canals. The father of modern dentistry, Pierre Fauchard, described a technique called "in tooth" in 1928. He used the watchmaker's reamer to prepare the canal after which a post fabricated from metal was fitted and secured in the canal. Richmond and Davis described different techniques for restorations which remained popular for a long time.

In the earlier days, a cast and post core crown used to be a single piece restoration. However, the trend today is to make two separate portions, i.e. post and core together cemented into the canal after which a crown is fabricated and cemented over it. The advantages of such a procedure include:

1. Easier to handle the wax patterns separately.
2. The expansion rates of the two castings may be controlled individually ensuring a better marginal fit.
3. Makes it possible to achieve ferrule effect. This is the binding of remaining tooth structure together and is obtained when the axial wall of the crown is placed apical to the missing tooth structure.
4. If the crown is to be replaced for some reason, the same is possible without the need to remove the post.
5. Different paths of insertion may be selected for the post and crown. This saves tooth structure.
6. When the tooth is part of an FPD, the path of insertion is controlled better by shaping of the core.

The materials and techniques have evolved over a period of years to its current form. A detail discussion of the same is made in the following sections.

Components of the Post Crown System

1. *The post:* It is highly rigid part accurately fits into the prepared root canal of the tooth.
2. *The core:* It is that part inserted in the pulp chamber which rebuilds the lost part of the coronal tooth structure.
3. *The extracoronal restoration:* It is that part restoring both esthetics and function of the tooth (Fig. 4.1).

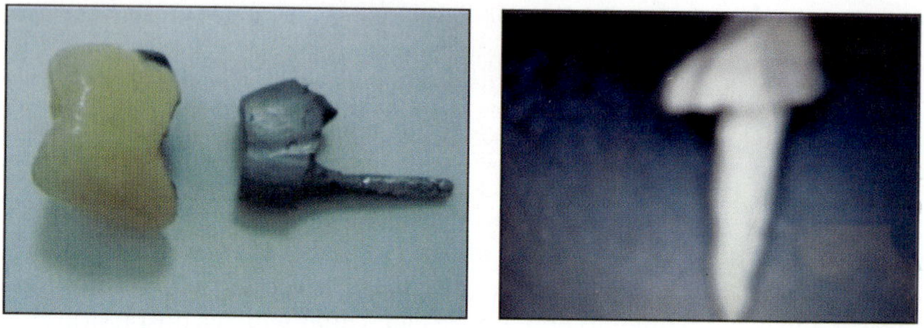

Fig. 4.1: Cast metallic post and core with the separate metal-ceramic crown.

The post and core are discussed in detail in the following sections while a discussion of the extracoronal restoration may be found in the chapter on principles of tooth preparation with individual tooth preparations.

THE POST

A post is that portion of the post and core restoration that fits and is cemented into the prepared root canal. A post and core crown is defined as a restoration in which the crown and cast post is one unit.

Classification of Posts

1. According to the Material

a. *All metallic*: The post and core are cast as a single piece.
b. *Combination of metal and non-metal:* This type could be either:
   1. Metallic post crown with non-metallic veneer.
   2. The post constructed from metal and the core from non-metal
c. *All non-metallic*: Recently introduced materials, such as zirconium oxide ceramic posts, and carbon fiber, glass fiber posts in combination with plastic core materials.

2. According to Manufacture

a. *Custom-cast posts:* These are custom made to fit into a prepared canal using elaborate lab procedures.

b. *Prefabricated posts*
- Posts with passive retention
- Posts with active retention.

Custom-cast Posts

Advantages

1. Close conformation to the configuration of the prepared canal.
2. Can be used in all cases of post and core restorations.
3. Are adaptable to large, irregularly shaped canals and orifices.
4. Can be adapted to be used with wrought posts and prefabricated plastic patterns.
5. Are strong.
6. Have considerable documentation to support their effectiveness.

Disadvantages

1. Lengthy procedure requires two appointments.
2. Expensive.
3. Less retentive.
4. Temporization between appointments is difficult.
5. Corrosion is a problem either due to casting defects or use of dissimilar alloys.
6. Risk of casting defects.
7. They may require the removal of additional tooth structure.

Prefabricated Posts

Advantages

1. They are relatively simple to use.
2. Less time consuming.
3. Completed in one appointment.
4. They are easy to temporize.
5. Cost effective.
6. Strong.

Disadvantages

1. Root has to be designed according to the post.
2. Cannot be used when considerable tooth structure is lost.
3. When the post and core are of different metals, corrosion may occur.
4. When attachments are required for a removable prosthesis, a separate casting has to be fabricated and cemented over it and cannot be attached to the post-core.

Preparation of the Post Space

When the decision to place a post is made even before the RCT, it is possible that only the apical 1/3rd of the canal be sealed with root canal filling material. However, it is better to completely fill the canal and then remove the coronal 2/3rds for the post space to ensure effective sealing of the lateral canals that might be present. When silver points are used to fill the canal, these must be removed and the canal retreated with gutta-percha.

The filling material may be removed by: Endodontic plugger.

Warmed Endodontic Plugger

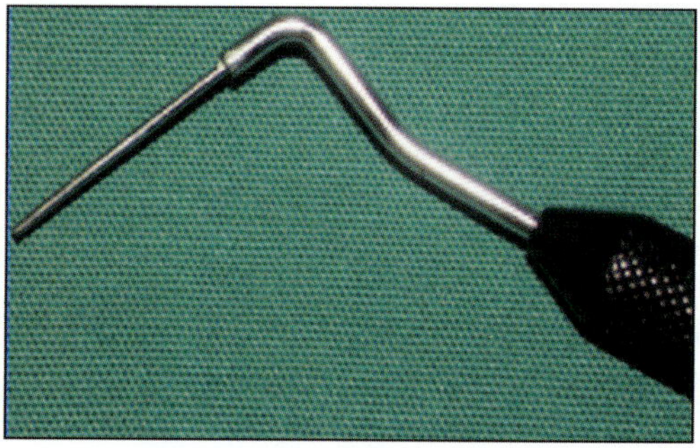

Fig. 4.2: Endodontic plugger

Advantages

- Reduces the possibility of dentin damage.
- Can be used immediately after obturation when the clinician is familiar with the root canal anatomy.
- Long history of successful use.
- Does not disturb the apical seal.

Disadvantages

- Time consuming.
- Difficult to use when the gutta-percha is old and has lost its elasticity.

Rotary Instrument With or Without Chemical Agents

Advantages

- Fast
- Can be used in old fillings.

Disadvantages:

- Cannot be used immediately after filling as it might disturb the apical seal.[4]

- Risk of dentin perforation.
- Cost of equipment.

Steps in Preparation of Post Space

1. Apply rubber dam.
2. Select an endodontic condenser which is large enough to hold the heat but without binding against the canal walls.
3. Determine the appropriate length of the post, i.e. working length minus 5 mm apical seal. In case of short teeth an absolute minimum of 3 mm apical filling should be left to maintain the seal. If it is not possible to achieve this without compromising on the minimum required post length, then the prognosis of such teeth is seriously impaired.
4. Mark the length on the instrument, heat it and place it in the canal to soften the gutta-percha. The filling is then removed gradually.
5. When using a rotary instrument, choose one that is slightly narrower than the canal. Special post preparation instruments like the Peeso-Reamers and Gates Glidden drills are used. These are considered safe tip instruments. The friction generated between the instrument and the filling is enough to soften the filling material and allows the rotary instrument to track the canal.
6. Once the gutta-percha is removed till the required depth, the canal is enlarged and shaped as required with an endodontic hand instrument or a low speed drill. A choice of the type or post is usually made before further preparation and then the canal is enlarged accordingly (Figs 4.3 and 4.4).

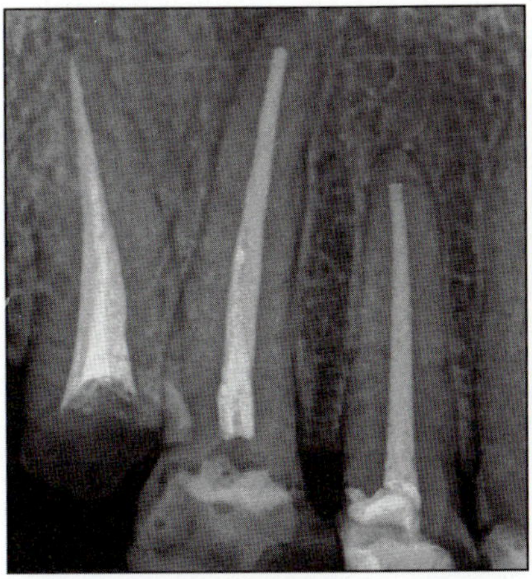

Fig. 4.3: Teeth with endodontic filling

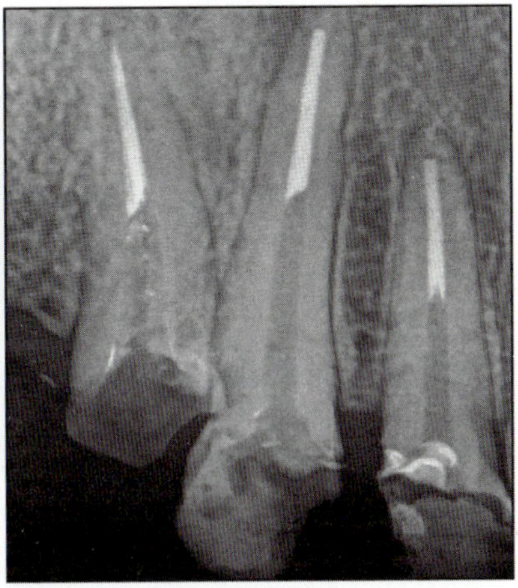

Fig. 4.4: Teeth with prepared post spaces

7. *Custom-made posts:* Often very little preparation is required. The canal is usually enlarged to 2 or 3 sizes higher than the last file size while simultaneously removing the undercuts. Care must be taken not to perforate the canals when additional shaping is done (Fig. 4.5).

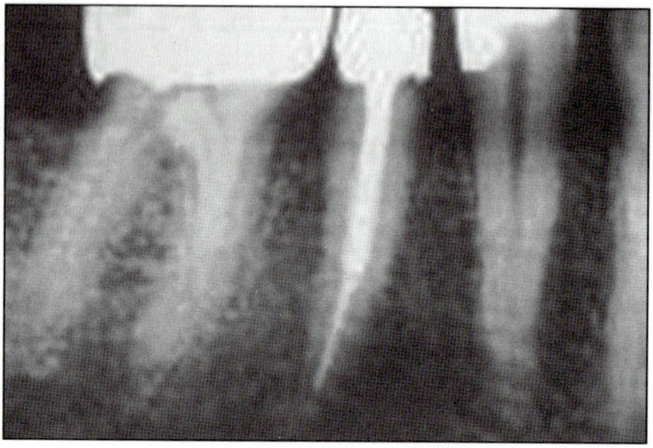

Fig. 4.5: Custom post in position

8. *Prefabricated posts*: The canal is enlarged to conform to the shape of the post chosen. Hand or rotary instruments may be used. A threaded post might require the use of a tap that prethreads the canal walls. It is better to use prefabricated posts that match standard endodontic instruments. Details may be found under the discussion of individual prefabricated posts (Fig. 4.6).

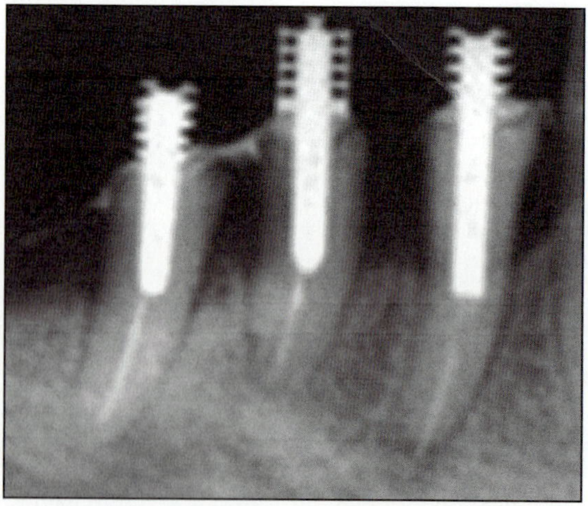

Fig. 4.6: Prefabricated posts in position

PRINCIPLES OF TOOTH PREPARATION

A. Conservation of Tooth Structure

I. Root Canal

- Only minimal tooth structure should be removed from the canal.
- Experimental testing of different post diameters showed that teeth with thicker posts fractured more easily than thinner posts (Fig. 4.7).[5]

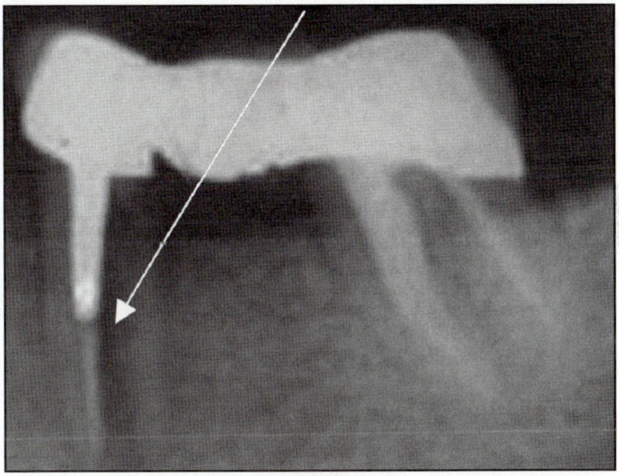

Fig. 4.7: Fracture line originating at the end of the post

- The roots are usually elongated faciolingually and have proximal developmental grooves. When the tooth is thinned, root fractures originate from these concavities[6]. Hence, uniform enlargement of the canal is not recommended (Fig. 4.8).

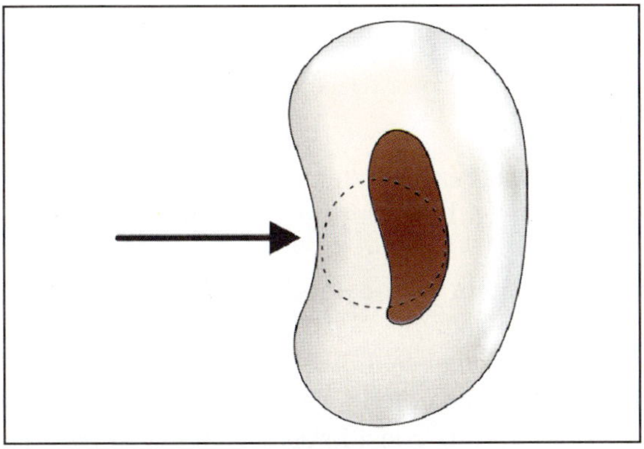

Fig. 4.8: Fracture lines may originate from proximal concavities

- Usually, one or two additional file sizes beyond the final file used for endodontic treatment are all that is essential.
- The enlargement should be enough if it enables the post to fit accurately and passively in the canal.

II. Crown

- Preserve as much of the crown as possible, as this helps reduce stress concentrations at the gingival margin and is the factor that decides clinical success.[7]
- Place the finish line on sound tooth structure to prevent fracture during function (ferrule) (Fig. 4.9).[8,9]

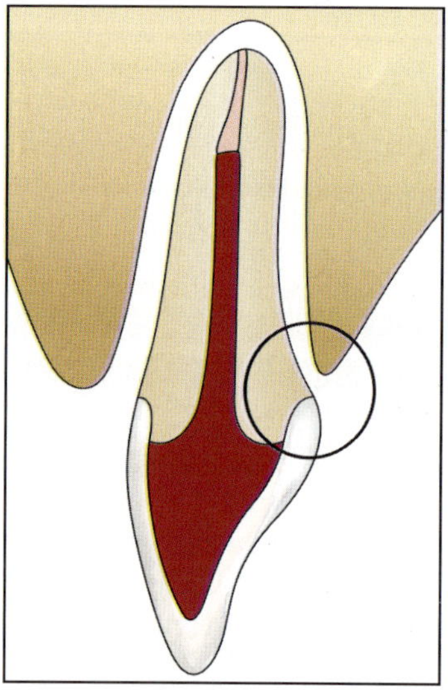

Fig. 4.9: Crown margins on sound tooth for ferrule

B. Obtaining Retention

I. Embedment Depth

- As the post length increases, retention increases.[10,11]
- The post should be as long as possible without disturbing the apical seal.
- Tooth length, canal morphology and root diameter in the apical 1/3rd should be taken into account.
- About 5 mm of the apical seal is left undisturbed.
- When the clinician is presented with a short root and tall clinical crown, an apical seal of 3 mm is considered acceptable (Fig. 4.10).

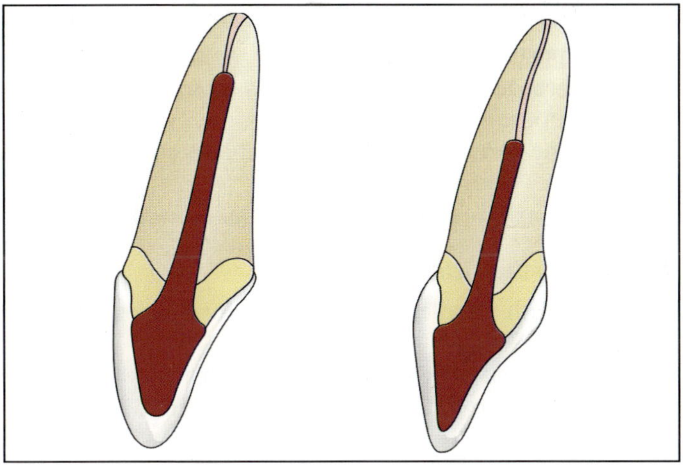

Fig. 4.10: Post extending till 5 mm short of apex is better compared to a shorter post

II. Post Diameter

- Since posts are not placed in perfect cylindrical channels, diameter makes a little difference in retentive capacity.
- Increasing the diameter of posts decreases the thickness of dentin that is available for stress distribution making the tooth highly susceptible to fracture.
- Post diameter that does not exceed 1/3rd of the cross-sectional diameter of the root is recommended (Fig. 4.11).

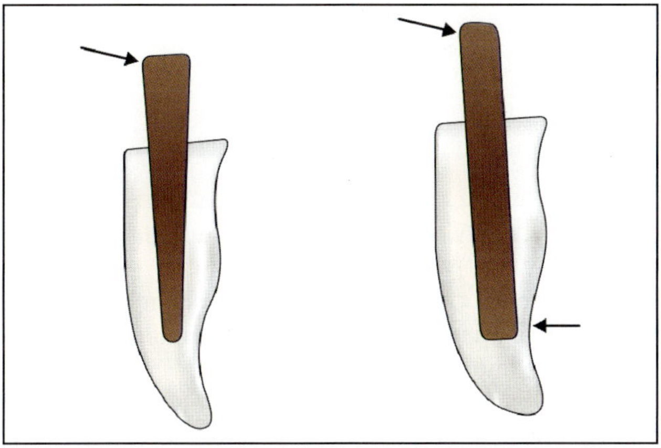

Fig. 4.11: Excessive thick post leads to weakening of tooth

III. Surface Morphology of the Posts

- A variety of post designs are available.
- A serrated, threaded or roughened post is more retentive compared to smooth-sided post.[12]
- Roughening the surfaces of the root canal also considerably increases retention.[13]
- Parallel-sided posts are more retentive than tapered posts.

IV. Geometry of the Canal

- Preparations with parallel walls and minimal taper have maximum retention.
- Elliptical cross-section of the roots dictate that they be prepared with minimal taper of 6 to 8 degrees to improve retention.

V. Number of Posts

- Increasing the number of posts is an option in the posterior teeth that have more than one root (Fig. 4.12).

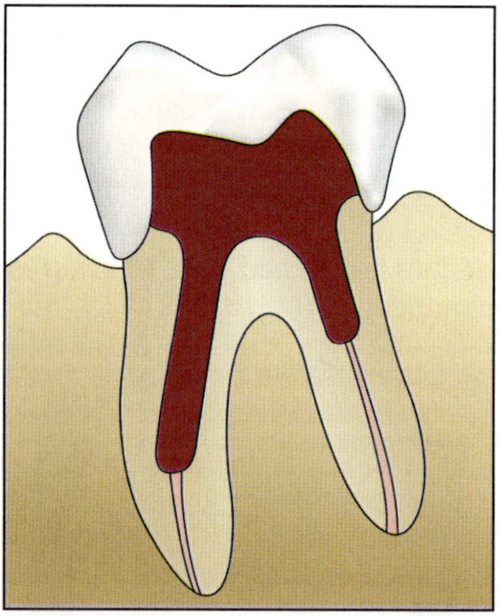

Fig. 4.12: Two posts placed in mandibular molar

- Usually the largest root is used for major post and the other roots will hold short auxiliary post, e.g. distal root of mandibular molar and palatal root of maxillary molar.
- The posts may be designed to have different paths of insertion to help in conservation of tooth structure. In such a case, the cast core and posts are casted in different portions and then cemented into position (Figs 4.13 and 4.14).

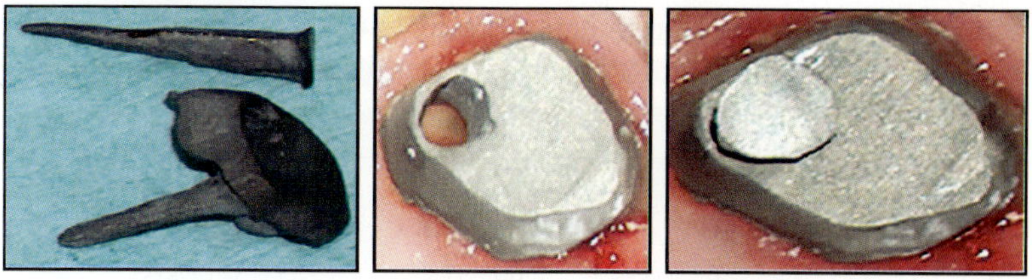

(a) (b) (c)

Fig. 4.13: The posts cast as two separate pieces and cemented together

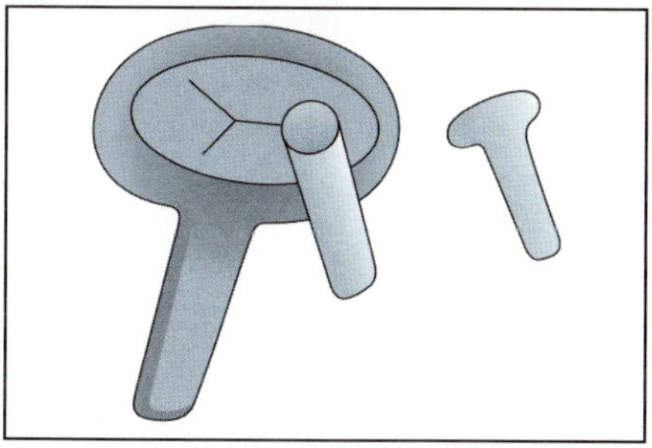

Fig. 4.14: Schematic drawing that represents final position of auxiliary post

VI. Cement Type

- Traditionally, zinc phosphate was the cement of choice. It has a little effect on retention.
- However, removing the smear layer to open the dentinal tubules so that the cementing medium may flow and lock into these tubules helps improve retention.
- 2.5 cc irrigation with 17% EDTA (7.5 pH) to chelate the calcium or phosphate salts from the dentin followed by 2.5 cc of 5.25% NaOCl to flush away the remaining decalcified dentin or organic material is used.
- Use of dentin bonding agents has been shown to improve retention.
- These are especially useful in cases of short posts and little retention.
- However, the luting agent must not be used to compensate for poor preparation design and ill-fitting post.

C. Obtaining Resistance

I. Resistance to Fracture

- The tooth resists fracture when the load on it is distributed over a large surface area rather than concentrating it in one area.

- Greater the thickness of remaining dentin, better is the stress distribution. As much dentin should be conserved as possible specially at the shoulder and apex.

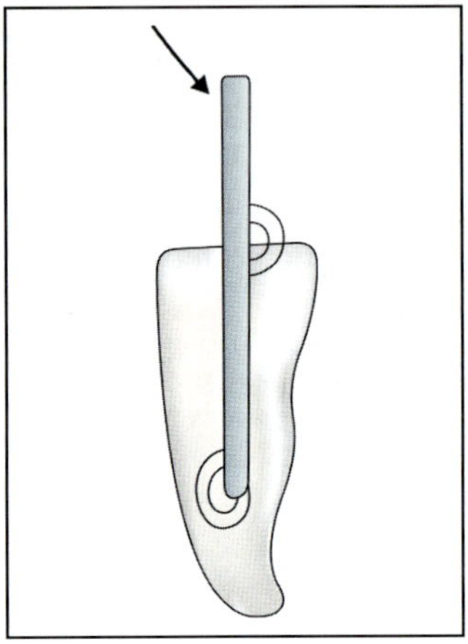

Fig. 4.15

- Greater the length of the post, greater is the stress distribution.
- Sharp angles act as areas of stress concentration and should be avoided.
- Parallel-sided posts distribute stress better than tapered posts which act as wedge.
- During cementation, a vent should be provided for the cement to escape to minimize stress build up.
- Threaded posts should be backed off a half turn to enable them to evenly distribute stress.[14]
- The cement layer contributes to stress distribution and should be of even thickness.

II. Resistance to Rotation

- In case of multiple posts, the auxiliary posts prevent rotation.
- When adequate coronal dentin remains, the vertical walls of the crown prevent rotation.
- In case of a single cylindrical post, an anti-rotation feature is incorporated by forming an extension into dentin in the coronal part of the post (Fig. 4.16).

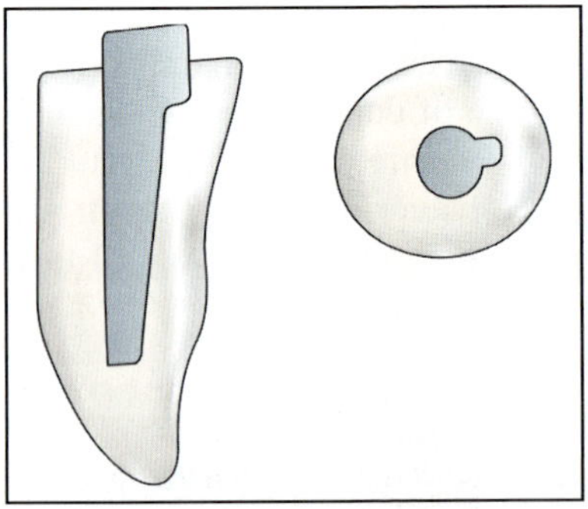

Fig. 4.16: Vertical and cross section of anti-rotation groove

FABRICATION OF CAST POSTS

The cast posts may be fabricated using two different techniques. A direct technique is recommended for single canals, whereas indirect procedure is more appropriate for multiple canals.

Direct Method

a. Direct Resin Pattern

- Lightly lubricate the canal.
- Select suitable plastic dowel to fit loosely in the canal, it should extend to the full depth of the prepared canal.
- Notches are prepared on the dowel surface to produce mechanical interlocking between the dowel and the resin.
- The self-curing resin is mixed to a thin consistency in a dappen dish.
- Fill the canal with the resin by the help of the plastic dowel which is previously coated with monomer.
- The coated dowel is seated into the canal.
- As the resin begins to stiffen, the plastic dowel is grasped by its end and the pattern is moved slightly in and out of the canal. This prevents the resin from being locked into the minute undercuts inside the canal.
- Once the resin has polymerized, remove the pattern.
- Check the apical part of the pattern by adding additional resin and reseating and removing the post, taking care not to lock it in the canal.
- Additional resin is added for the core build up.
- Complete the coronal preparation (Fig. 4.17).

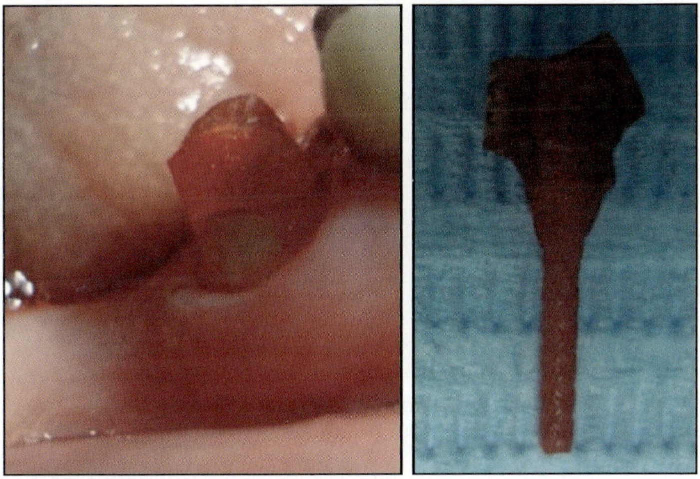

Fig. 4.17: Direct pattern prepared in the mouth

b. Readymade Plastic Burnout Post

- After preparation of the root canals with special drills, select the readymade plastic pattern having the same shape and size of the drill to fit properly and accurately inside the canal.
- Build up wax or resin for the core.

Indirect Technique

- This technique involves making impressions of the prepared root canals along with the coronal tooth structure after which the post and core are fabricated in the laboratory.
- Select a serrated stainless steel wire to fit loosely inside the canal and extend to the full length of the space.
- Tissue displacement of the surrounding gingiva is performed.
- Using the special syringe, inject the canal with elastomeric impression material.
- Seat the wire reinforcement to the full depth of the post space.
- Put more impression material around the prepared tooth and insert the previously filled tray.
- Remove the tray, evaluate it and pour the final cast (Fig. 4.18).

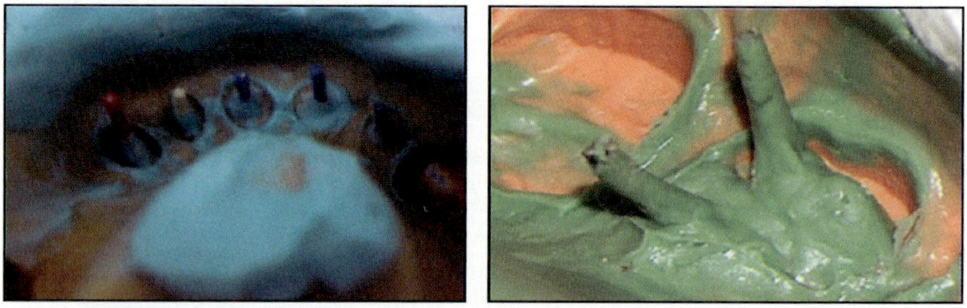

Fig. 4.18: Impressions of the prepared post space made with addition silicone

- Once the cast is obtained, lubricate the post space with die lubricant.
- Wax or resin is used to fabricate the post and core on the cast which is then casted in metal and cemented onto the prepared tooth.

PREFABRICATED POSTS

- Posts are supplied in different sizes, designs, and shapes.
- The majority of the prefabricated posts are designed to be matched with special drills or endodontic files for root canal preparation before post insertion.

Classification of Prefabricated Posts

A-Tapered, smooth-sided posts.
B- Tapered, serrated posts.
C- Tapered, threaded posts.
D- Parallel, smooth-sided posts.
E- Parallel, serrated posts.
F- Parallel, threaded posts.

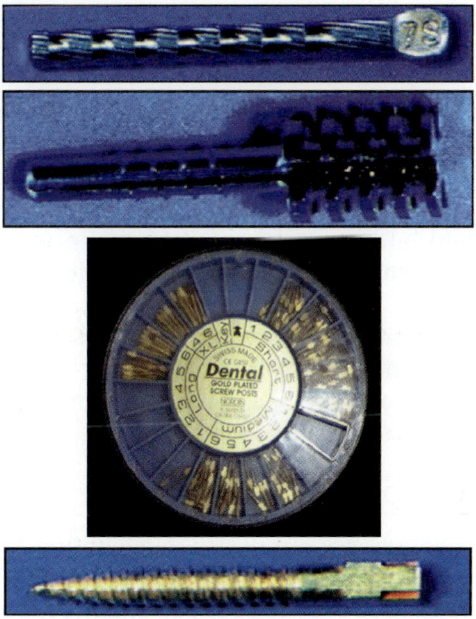

Fig. 4.19: Different types of prefabricated posts

THE CORE

The core of a post and core restoration replaces missing tooth structure, and forms the shape of the tooth preparation.

Core Fabrication

Core for Cast Posts

- It can be shaped in resin or wax and added to the post pattern before the assembly is cast in metal.
- This prevents possible failure at the post-core interface.

Core for Preformed Posts

- The cores may be cast onto preformed posts but this may lead to alteration of its physical properties.
- The core could be formed with restorative materials such as amalgam, reinforced glass ionomer or composite resin.
- The *advantages* of these materials as core build up are:
  - Maximum conservation of tooth structure because the undercuts are not to be removed.
  - Treatment is complete in one appointment, less patient visit.
  - There are fewer laboratory procedures, i.e. no casting of core onto post.
  - Good strength characteristic due to good adaptation to tooth structure.
- The *disadvantages* of these materials as core build up are:
  - Corrosion of amalgam cores, low tensile strength of glass ionomer or continued polymerization and high coefficient of thermal expansion of composite cores may affect long-term success of the restoration.
  - Microleakage with thermocycling is found to be greater under composite and amalgam cores.
  - An operative procedure such as matrix application is difficult particularly on badly damaged teeth.

CEMENTATION OF POSTS

Most of the procedures are similar to cementation of crowns. The differences being

i. A lentulospiral is used to coat the canal with the cement.
ii. In parallel-sided posts, a vent is provided along the side of the post for the cement to escape and reduce pressure build up.

REFERENCES

1. Johnson J.K., et al. Evaluation and restoration of endodontically treated posterior teeth, *J Am Dent Assoc* 1976; 93:597.
2. Warren M.A., et al. *In vitro* comparison of bleaching agents on the crowns and roots of discolored teeth. *J Endodont* 1990;16: 463–7.
3. Sorenson J.A., Maritnoff J.T., Endodontically treated teeth as abutments. *J Prosthet Dent* 1985; 53: 631–6.
4. Dickey D.J., et al. Effect of post space preparation on apical seal using solvent techniques and peeso reamers. *J Endodont* 1982; 8: 351–4.
5. Helfer A.R., et al. Determination of the moisture content of vital and pulpless teeth. Oral surg 1972; 34: 661.
6. Felton D.A., Webb E.L., Kanoy B.E., Jay Dugoni. Threaded endodontic dowels: Effect of post design on incidence of root fracture. *J Prosthet Dent* 1991; 65: 179–187.

7. Henry P.J. Photoelastic analysis of post core restorations. *Aust. Dent. J* 1977; 22: 157–9.
8. Sorensen J.A., Engelman M.J. Ferrule design and fracture resistance of endodontically treated teeth. *J Prosthet. Dent* 1990; 63: 529–36.
9. Gegauff, A.G. Change in strength from creating a ferrul via crown-lengthening, *J Dent. Res* 1999; 78: 223–7.
10. Standlee J.P., Caputo A.A., Hanson E.C. Retention of endodontic dowels: effects of cement, dowel length, diameter and design. *J Prosthet Dent* 1978: 39: 401–5.
11. Kurer H.G., Combe E.C., Grant A.A. Factors influencing the retention of dowels. *J Prosthet Dent* 1977; 38: 515–25.
12. Ruemping DR, Lund MR, Schnell RJ. Retention of dowels subjected to tensile and torsional forces. *J Prosthet. Dent* 1979; 41: 159–162.
13. Wood W.W. Retention of posts in teeth with non-vital pulps. *J Prosthet. Dent* 1983; 49: 504–6.
14. Mendoza D.B., Eakle W.S. Retention of posts cemented with various dentinal bonding cements. *J Prosthet. Dent* 1994; 72: 591–4.

PART II

Parts of FPD

5

Abutments

Though, strictly not a part of the FPD, it is discussed here to provide continuity to the reader.

A tooth, a portion of a tooth, or that portion of a dental implant that supports and/or retains a prosthesis.

CRITERIA FOR ABUTMENT SELECTION

1. Bone Support/Periodontal Ligament Area

- *Ante's law:* The abutment teeth should have a combined pericemental area equal to or greater than the tooth or teeth to be replaced.
- Lesser the bone support, lessened is the capacity to serve as abutments.
- A ratio of 1:1 or greater would satisfy "Ante's law".
- Loss of periodontal support due to root resorption is less critical as compared to loss of alveolar crestal bone because of greater diameter of the root at the crest.
- Long edentulous span and lesser abutments would lead to:
  - i. Overstressing of periodontal ligament.
  - ii. Biomechanical factors (leverage and torque) and material failure

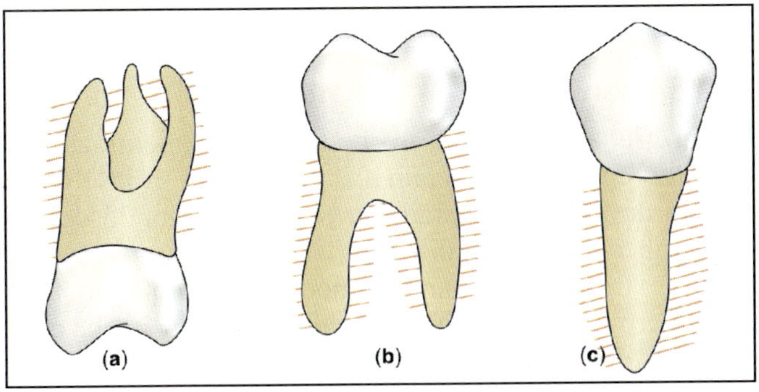

Fig. 5.1: Relative root surface areas shaded in red: (a) Maxillary molar, (b) Mandibular molar, (c) Mandibular premolar

2. Root Configuration and Angulations

- Roots that are broader labiolingually than they are mesiodistally are preferable to roots that are round in cross section.
- Multi-rooted posterior teeth with widely separated roots will offer better periodontal support than roots that converge, fuse or are conical.
- Conical roots can be used as satisfactory abutments for short span FPDs.
- When single rooted, those with evidence of irregular configuration or with some curvature in the apical third are preferable to perfectly tapered roots.
- Roots with developmental grooves are better as abutments.
- Teeth that are well aligned will provide better support than a tilted one as the forces are directed along their long axes (Fig. 5.2).

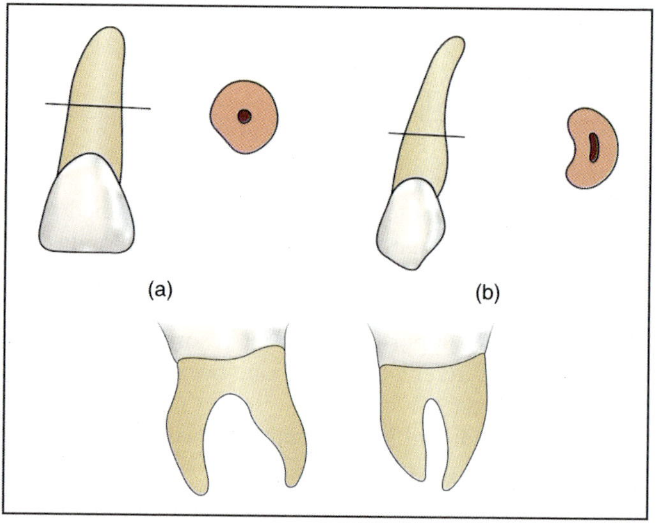

Fig. 5.2: (a) Round cross-section of maxillary incisor, (b) Wider labiolingually, mesial developmental groove, distal curvature in the apical third of root

3. Tooth Alignment

- Teeth that are well aligned are better as abutments as they allow convenient preparation to obtain a common path of insertion.
- If the teeth deviate from parallelism by more than 25 degrees, tooth preparation becomes more difficult.[1]
- In cases of extreme malalignment, modified tooth preparation like the mesial half crown or orthodontic uprighting[2,3] may be the only choice.
- The use of a dental surveyor is advocated in some cases to obtain a parallel path of insertion (Fig. 5.3).

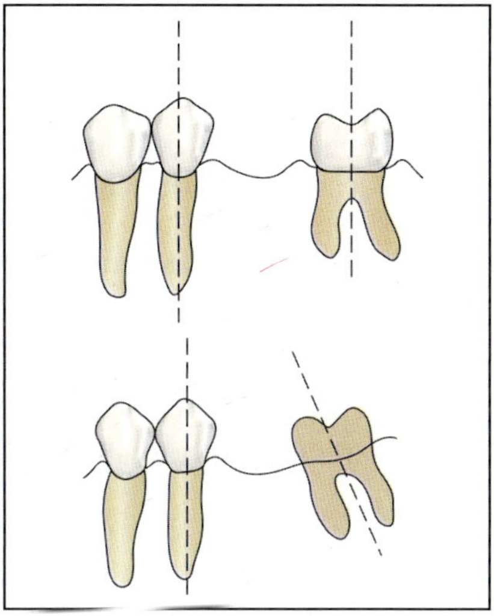

Fig. 5.3: Comparison of the alignment of abutments

4. Crown–Root Ratio

- It is the ratio of the length of tooth occlusal to the alveolar crest to that embedded in bone.
- An apical migration of crestal bone causes the lever arm of that portion out of bone to increase, in turn increasing chance for harmful lateral forces.
- Optimum ratio is 2:3.
- Minimum of 1:1 is acceptable under normal circumstances.
- Ratio greater than 1:1 might be considered adequate when the opposing occlusion is composed of artificial teeth or mobile, periodontally involved teeth.
- 1/3rd loss of crestal bone = loss of ½ support of PDL (Fig. 5.4).

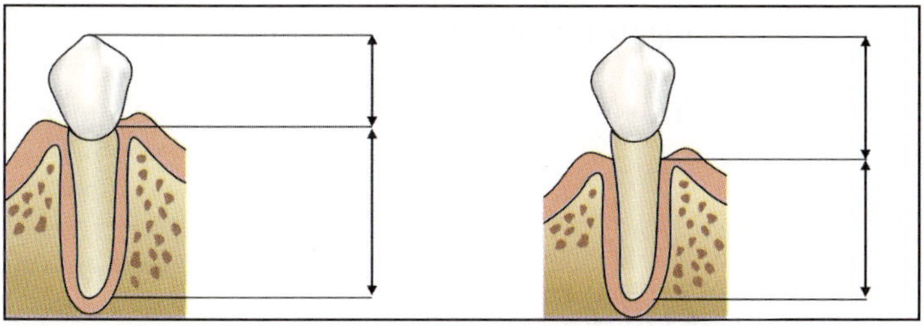

Fig. 5.4: Comparison of the altered crown to root ratios due to loss of crestal bone and gingival recession

5. Tooth Vitality

- Whenever possible, an abutment should be a vital tooth, however, an endodontically treated tooth, that is asymptomatic, with radiographic evidence of complete obturation and good seal, with some sound coronal structure present or that can be compensated by core restoration may be used.
- Teeth that have been pulp capped should not be used unless endodontically treated.
- Teeth with large existing restorations should be assessed under isolation after the restoration, cavity liners and residual caries are removed.
- Non-vital teeth are contraindicated as abutments for cantilevered FPDs.[4]

6. Supporting Tissues

- The supporting tissues should be healthy and free from inflammation.
- Inflamed tissues are placed more coronal and need to be brought back to health before a decision on margin placement can be made.
- Inflamed tissues are injured faster and tend to bleed making procedures like tooth preparation, tissue retraction and impression making difficult.

7. Available Tooth Structure and Crown Morphology

Influences Treatment Option

i. Intentional RCT may be necessary in extensive decay, large restorations, and fractures of teeth.
ii. In already RC treated teeth, a need for post and core may depend on this factor.[5]
iii. Partial veneer retainers are possible only in teeth with adequate labiolingual bulk.
iv. Crown lengthening to accommodate caries or pre-existing restoration may be required.
v. Resin-bonded retainers can be planned only when adequate enamel exists.

8. Selective Extraction

When Adjacent Teeth are Better Abutments

i. Sole remaining lower incisor and FPD planned between canines.
ii. Periodontally involved teeth that cannot be salvaged.

S.No.	Condition	Modification
1.	Bone loss from periodontal disease	Increase the number of abutments
2.	Changes in the axial inclination of teeth	Increase the number of abutments
3.	Migration of teeth with reduced edentulous span	Decrease the number of abutments
4.	Less favorable occlusal relation with increased forces	Increase the number of abutments
5.	Arch form that produces greater leverage forces	Increase the number of abutments
6.	Endo treated abutments with root resection	Increase the number of abutments
7.	Increased tooth mobility after osseous surgery	Increase the number of abutments

Table 5.1: Factors modifying the Ante's law

SPECIAL CONDITIONS

1. Periodontally Compromised Teeth as Abutments

- C:R > 1:1 have been successfully used as abutments.[6]
- Meticulous root planing during the active phase of the treatment, proper plaque control during the observation period and the occlusal design of the prosthesis contribute to their use as abutments.[7,8]
- The goal is to prevent any further increase in mobility.
- Patients need to be well motivated and highly proficient in plaque removal.

2. Pier Abutments

- An abutment with edentulous areas on either side is called a pier abutment (Fig. 5.5).

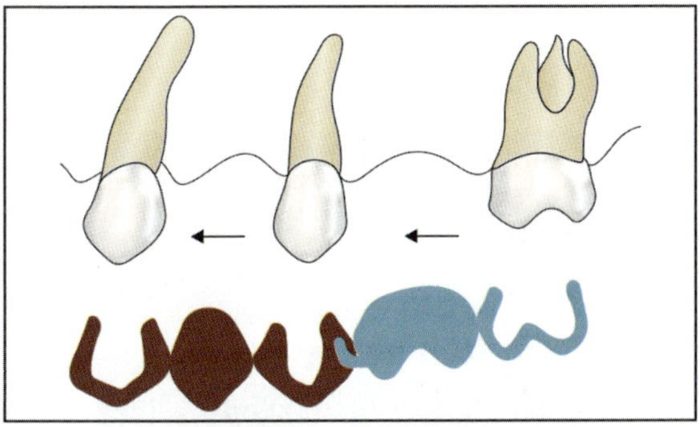

Fig. 5.5: Pier abutment—maxillary second premolar

- It has the potential to exert unseating force on terminal retainers.[9]
- Keyway on the distal side of pier abutments and key on the mesial of pontic causes firmer placement of the key into keyway during function.
- Susceptible to torque forces.

3. Cantilevered FPDs

- Pontic is attached to the retainer on one side only.
- Long-term prognosis is poor as cantilever will induce lateral forces and forces are best tolerated when directed along the long axis of the teeth. May lead to tipping, rotation or drifting of teeth.
  Applications today:
    i. Replacement of lateral incisor using canine
    ii. Multiple missing teeth are replaced
    iii. Implant supported prosthesis.

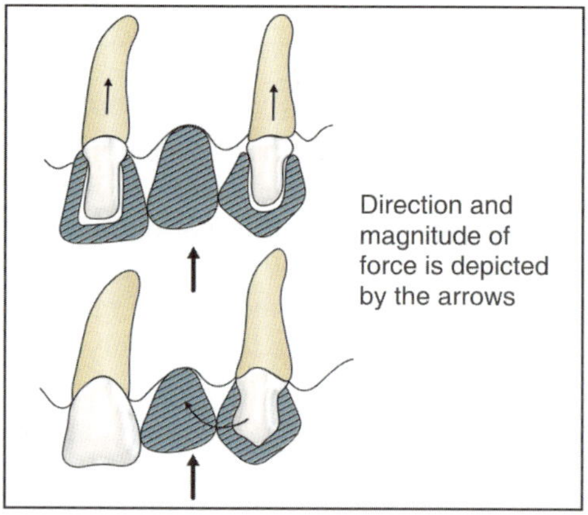

Fig. 5.6: Cantilevered maxillary lateral incisor

4. Mesially Tilted Second Molar

- Commonly seen condition.[10]

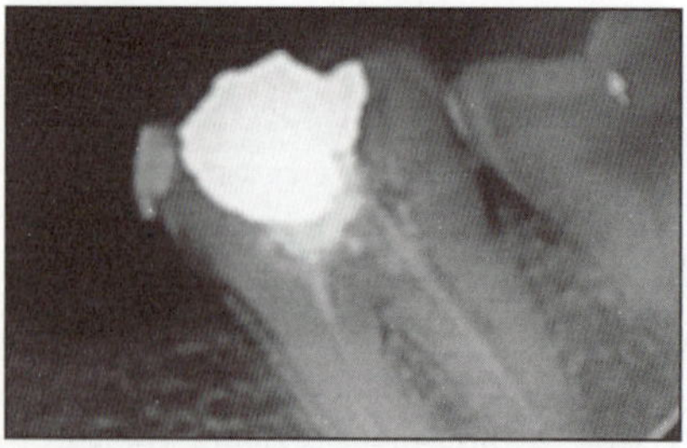

Fig. 5.7

- Positional relationship does not allow parallel path of insertion.
- Further complicated with eruption of third molar teeth.
- Treatment options
  i. Slight tilting—increased preparation of mesial surface of second molar and conventional FPD
  ii. Removal of third molar and orthodontic up righting of second molar.
  iii. Partial veneer preparation (Mesial half crown) on distal abutment, a split pontic or use of key and keyway attachments.

REFERENCES

1. Reynolds J.M. Abutment selection for fixed prosthodontics, *J Prosthet. Dent* 1968; 19: 483–8.
2. Khouw F.E., Norton L.A. The mechanism of fixed molar uprighting appliances. *J Prosthet. Dent* 1972; 27: 381–9.
3. Miller T.E., Orthodontic therapy for the restorative patient. I. Biomechanic aspects, *J Prosthet. Dent* 1989; 61: 268.
4. Schweitzer J.M., Schweitzer R.D., Schweitzer J. Free end pontics used on fixed partial dentures, *J Prosthet. Dent* 1968; 20: 120–38.
5. Shillingburg H.T., Jacobi R., Brackett S.E., Preparation modifications for damaged vital posterior teeth, *Dent clin North Am* 1985; 29: 305.
6. Freilich M.A., Breeding L.C., Keagle J.G., Garnick J.J. Fixed partial dentures supported by periodontally compromised teeth, *J Prosthet. Dent* 1991; 65: 607–11.
7. Nyman S., Ericsson I. The capacity of reduced periodontal tissues to support fixed bridgework, *J of Clin Periodontol.* 1982; 9: 409–414.
8. Nyman S., Lindhe J., Lundgren D., The role of occlusion for the stability of fixed bridges in patients with reduced periodontal tissue support. *J Clin Periodontol* 1975; 2: pp. 53–66.
9. Shillingburg H.T., Fisher D.W., Non-rigid connectors for fixed partial dentures. JADA, 1973; 87: 1195–9.
10. Picton DCA. Tilting movements of teeth during biting. *Arch Oral Boil* 1962; 7: 151–6.

6 Retainers

REQUIREMENTS

1. It should restore the anatomy of the abutment tooth.
2. Should not be harmful to adjacent tissues.
3. Should not harm esthetics.
4. Have adequate strength to withstand masticatory forces.
5. Maintain the tooth positions.
6. Have proper contact with adjacent teeth to prevent food lodgement
7. Should correct mild misalignments.
8. Improve masticatory efficiency.
9. Be easy to fabricate.

CLASSIFICATION OF RETAINERS

I. Based on Location

1. Intracoronal Retainers

- Modified Class II inlay and MOD onlay
- Pinledge retainers

2. Extracoronal Retainers

- Full veneer
- Partial veneer

3. Radicular Retainers

- Dowel crown
- Richmond crown
- Post and core restoration

II. Based on Material

1. Metal
2. Ceramic
3. Metal-ceramic

EXTRACORONAL RETAINERS

Partial Veneer Crowns

It is a restoration covering two or more surfaces of tooth usually being lingual, proximal, occlusal or incisal except the buccal or labial surface.

Indications

1. Coronal tooth structure is intact/minimally restored; with intact buccal wall.
2. Teeth with crown size that is average or that exceeds the average.
3. Teeth with normal crown anatomy, i.e. without excess cervical constrictions.
4. Anterior teeth with adequate labiolingual thickness.
5. Teeth with reasonably good axial alignment.
6. Cases of short edentulous span.
7. Expected occlusal forces are average or less.
8. When alteration of the occlusal surface is needed.

Contraindications

1. High caries index—the increased margin to finish line interface are susceptible to decay.
2. Teeth with short clinical crown due to the inability to gain adequate retention and resistance form.
3. Teeth with extensive core restorations. The unveneered surface should be supported by sound tooth structure for adequate strength and this is not possible in heavily restored teeth.
4. Teeth with deep cervical abrasion—it is difficult to establish finish line. A complete crown is indicated as it minimizes sensitivity.
5. Teeth with severe cervical constriction—as they require excessive axial reduction to provide adequate groove length thus jeopardizing the pulp health.
6. Thin teeth—as there is inadequate tooth structure to place grooves and existent fear of undermining the facial enamel.
7. Cases of long span FPD—higher chances of dislodgement.
8. Endodontically treated teeth, because insufficient supporting tooth structure remains for the retentive features.
9. Dentition with active periodontal disease.
10. Poorly aligned abutment teeth, because problems with unsupported enamel often result.

Advantages

1. Conservation of tooth structure as a few surfaces are left intact.
2. Better esthetics—as facial enamel is retained.

3. Reduced pulpal and periodontal damage during tooth preparation.
4. Margins may be placed supragingival thus increasing biocompatibility with supporting tissues.
5. Margins are easily polished because of improved access.
6. Margins are easily accessible to oral hygiene maintenance.
7. The luting cement can escape more easily promoting an easy complete seating of the casting.
8. Because of direct visibility, verification of seating and cement removal are simple.
9. The intact tooth structure permits electric pulp testing.

Disadvantages

1. Less retentive compared to complete veneer crown.
2. Preparation is difficult, because only limited adjustments can be made in the path of withdrawal.
3. Some metal may be displayed which may be esthetically unacceptable.
4. Preparation is limited to fairly intact teeth, average in size and normally shaped.
5. Proximally bulbous teeth pose the danger of leaving unsupported enamel.

Types of Partial Veneer Retainers

I. Posterior Teeth

a. Three-quarter or 3/4th crown.
b. Reverse 3/4th crown.
c. Modified 3/4th or Mesial half crown or Kennedy Carmichael crown.
d. 7/8th crown.

II. Anterior Teeth

a. 3/4th crown
b. 3/4th crown with Pinledges
c. Pinledges.

Three-quarter crown (Fig. 6.1)

- Facial surface is left intact.

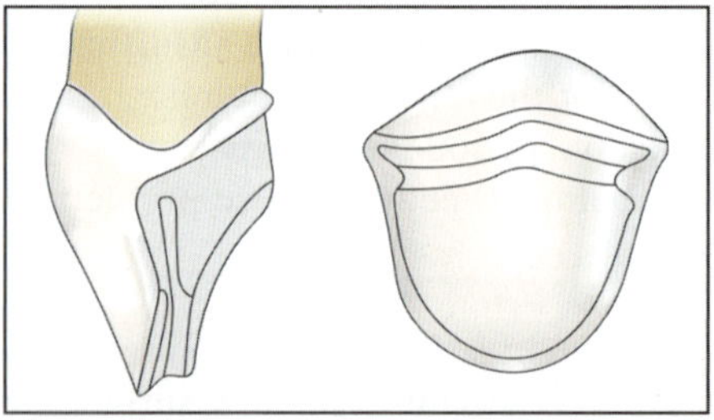

Fig. 6.1: 3/4th Crown on maxillary premolar

- Only a bevel extends beyond the bucco-occlusal or incisolabial line angle.
- In the anterior teeth, the preparation may be combined with pinledges for increased retention.

Reverse 3/4th crown

- Indicated on mandibular molars with severe lingual inclination.
- The buccal surface is prepared while the lingual surface is left intact.
- This crown is not applicable in the maxillary arch.

7/8th crown (Fig. 6.2)

- Generally indicated for maxillary molars that are sound mesially but have extensive carious involvement or a previous restoration on the distal surface.
- The crown preparation extends the finish line to the mid facial surface, avoiding an unnecessary display of metal on the mesial surface.

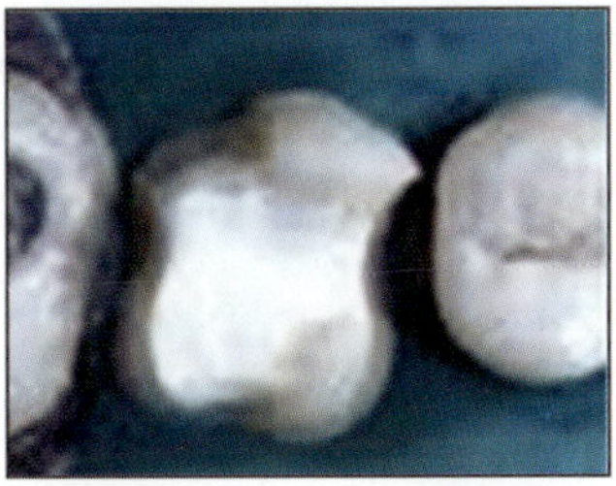

Fig. 6.2: Maxillary first molar prepared for 7/8th crown

Mesial 1/2 crown (Fig. 6.3)

- Indicated for a mesially tilted molar tooth.
- Covers all surfaces except the distal surface.

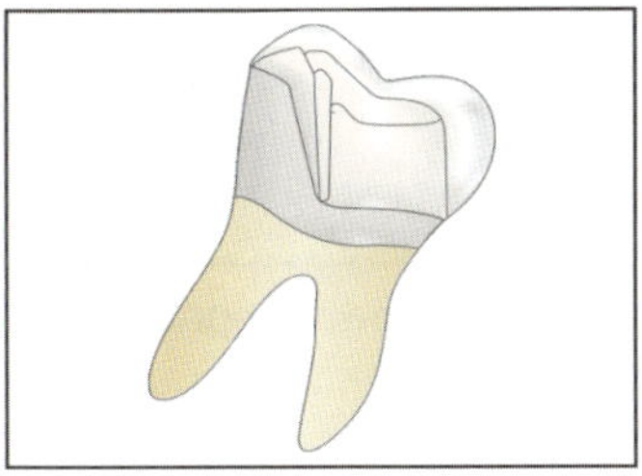

Fig. 6.3: Mesial 1/2 crown on tilted mandibular molar

- Especially useful when a tilted molar is to be used as an abutment for FPD.

Full Veneer Crowns

General indications

1. Situations that demand maximum retention and resistance form.
2. Short abutment teeth where high displacement forces are anticipated.
3. Long edentulous span to maximize retention.
4. When all surface of the teeth need to be covered either due to decalcification or caries/modification of occlusion.
5. Previous full veneer crown.
6. Poor abutment alignment to improve contours.

Contraindications

1. Poor oral hygiene.
2. When a more conservative preparation can be used (when intact buccal or lingual wall remains).
3. Active untreated periodontal disease.

TYPES

1. Complete cast crown restoration/full metal crown.
2. Metal-ceramic crown.
3. All ceramic crowns.
4. Acrylic fused to metal crowns.
5. Composite fused to metal crowns.

Full Metal Veneer Crown

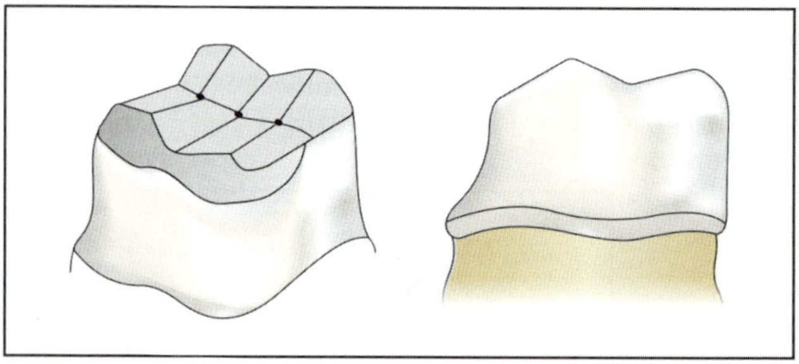

Fig. 6.4: Full metal veneer crown preparation in mandibular arch

Indications

1. Teeth that exhibit extensive coronal destruction either by caries or trauma.
2. Any posterior teeth in the non-esthetic zone.
3. Endodontically treated abutment teeth.

4. When correction of axial contours is not possible with a more conservative preparation.
5. When the restoration is to support a removable partial denture. (Makes provision for proper axial contours and houses the occlusal rests.)
6. Occlusal forces are greater than average.

Contraindications

1. When a high esthetic need exists.
2. If adequate axial contours exist or can be obtained with slight enamel modification.

Advantages

1. It imparts strength to the teeth as it compensates for the loss of tooth structure.
2. Has greater resistance and retention form compared to partial veneer.
3. Axial contours and contacts can be conveniently developed.
4. Protects the coronal structure compromised by extensive caries or restoration.

Disadvantages

1. Unaesthetic hence restricted to posterior.
2. Non-conservative of tooth structure.
3. Preparation causes extensive pulpal and periodontal insult.
4. Extensive involvement of supporting tissues.
5. Arduous preparation procedure.
6. After cementation, vitality testing is no longer feasible.
7. Caries under the restoration is difficult to detect.

Tooth reduction guidelines

- Centric or functional cusps: 1.5 mm with bevel of 45 degrees.
- Non-centric cusps: 1 mm
- Axial reduction or chamfer width: 0.5 mm.

Porcelain Fused to Metal Crowns

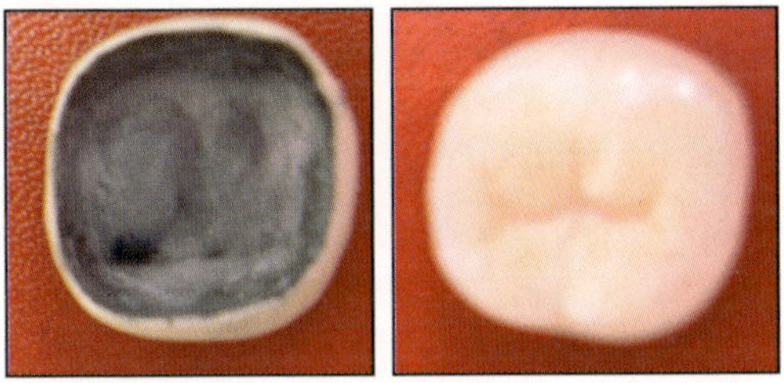

Cementing surface Occlusal surface

Fig. 6.5

Indications

1. Teeth in esthetic area that require complete coverage.
2. When the crown needs to incorporate rest seats, milled proximal and reciprocal guide plane to support an RPD. (These are incorporated in the metal part of the crown.)
3. Patients with reduced inter-occlusal clearance and a strong masticatory musculature.
4. Endodontically treated teeth.

Contraindications

1. In young patient with large pulp chambers.
2. When esthetics is not a concern.

Advantages

1. Combines the strength of metal with the esthetics of all ceramic crowns.
2. Good retention and resistance form.
3. Permits correction of axial contours.
4. Preparation is less demanding compared to partial veneer retainers.
5. Strength imparted to the tooth.
6. Can be used in high stress situations.
7. Better marginal fit compared to all ceramic.

Disadvantages

1. Non-conservative of tooth structure.
2. Requirement of subgingival margins for esthetics, increases risk of periodontal disease.[1,2]
3. Inferior esthetics compared to all ceramic restorations
4. Technique sensitive designing and fabrications.
5. Expensive.
6. Difficult to obtain accurate occlusion in porcelain.

Tooth reduction guidelines

1. Incisal reduction—2 mm
2. Occlusal reduction—1.5 mm (since esthetics is not as critical).
3. Labial or buccal reduction—1.2 to 1.5 mm.
4. Other axial reduction with chamfer width—0.5 mm.

All-ceramic Crowns (Fig. 6.6)

Indications

1. Areas of high esthetic requirement.

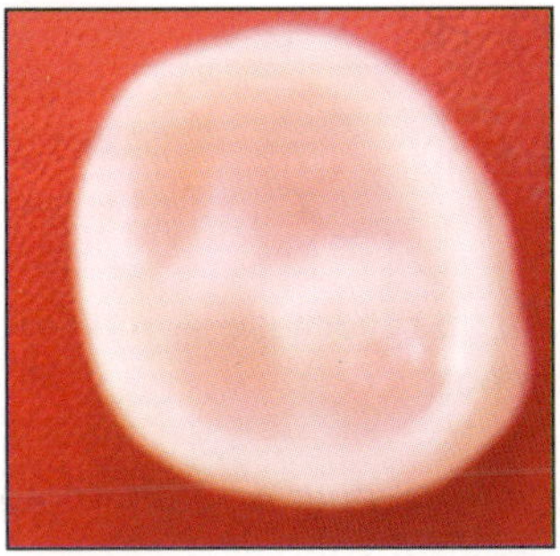

Fig. 6.6: All-ceramic crown—tissue surface

2. Relatively intact teeth with sufficient coronal structure to support the restoration (specially in incisal area, where porcelain should not exceed 2 mm thickness).
3. Areas with a favorable distribution of occlusal load.

Contraindications

1. When occlusal loading is not favorable.
2. When tooth structure is not adequate to provide an even width of 1mm circumferentially.
3. Areas of high stress.
4. Edentulous span more than one missing posterior tooth.

Advantages

1. Superior esthetics.
2. Good tissue response even for subgingival margin.
3. More conservative reduction of facial surface compared to metal ceramic crown.

Disadvantages

1. Reduced strength compared to metal ceramic crowns.
2. Requires a shoulder finish line along the circumference, for adequate support.
3. Proximal and lingual reduction is less conservative than those needed for metal ceramic crown.
4. Difficult to obtain close fitting margins with porcelain.
5. Incisal edge should be adequately supported by tooth to avoid brittle fracture.
6. Cannot be used in high stress posterior partial edentulous condition.
7. Large connectors impinge on interdental papilla.
8. Wear of opposing natural dentition.
9. Use restricted to 3 unit bridges only.

INTRACORONAL RETAINERS

Inlays and Onlays (Metal)

Indications

1. Small carious lesion in an otherwise sound tooth.
2. Adequate dentinal support.
3. Low caries rate.
4. Tooth replacement not exceeding a single tooth.
5. Normal or minimal occlusal stresses.
6. Abutments in good alignment.
7. Onlays are used when a damaged occlusal surface needs to be restored with a casting.
8. Onlays are indicated is severely worn dentition.

Contraindications

1. Tooth with insufficient bulk to provide resistance and retention form.
2. Caries or existing restorations that extend beyond the facial or lingual line angles.
3. High caries index.
4. Poor plaque control.
5. Poor dentinal support.
6. Heavy occlusal stress.

Advantages

1. Conserves tooth structure.
2. When accurately cast and finished, they do not deteriorate.
3. Noble metals do not corrode or causes discoloration.
4. Inexpensive.
5. Onlays reduce risk of tooth fracture.

Disadvantages

1. In restoration of a small carious lesion it is not very conservative of tooth structure, additional tooth removal is necessary to achieve a cavity preparation without undercuts.
2. MOD inlays increase the risk of cusp fracture.
3. Rely on bulk tooth for resistance and retention form.
4. Display of metal
5. Cannot be used in areas of high stress.
6. Increased finish line exposure.

Ceramic Inlays and Onlays (Fig. 6.7)

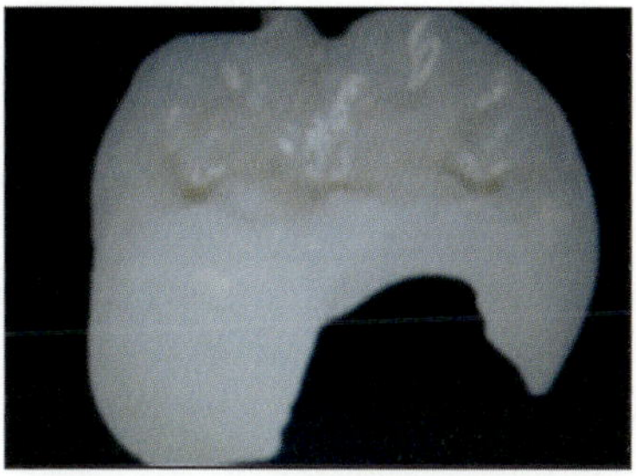

Fig. 6.7: Ceramic inlays and onlays

Indications

1. High demand for esthetics.
2. Low caries rate.
3. Intact buccal and lingual enamel.

Contraindications

1. Poor oral hygienic.
2. Active caries.
3. Excessive occlusal loading expected.

Advantages

1. Superior esthetics.
2. Conservative preparation and enable most of the remaining enamel to be preserved.
3. Durability.
4. Marginal leakage is reduced as the luting layer of resin is very thin.

Disadvantages

1. Time consuming.
2. Expensive
3. Accurate occlusion is difficult to achieve.
4. Intraoral occlusal adjustment is impractical because they are fragile.
5. Abrasion of opposing dentition.
6. Wear of luting agents can lead to marginal gaps and further chipping or caries.
7. Finishing of margins is difficult in less accessible areas.
8. Resin flash or overhangs are difficult to detect and can initiate periodontal disease.
9. Longevity questionable.

Pinledge Retainers

A pinledge retainer can be used as a single restoration to establish guidance or as a retainer for a FPD or to splint periodontally compromised teeth. Retention and resistance are provided primarily by pins that extend 2 mm into the dentin.

Indications

1. Undamaged anterior teeth in dentitions with a low caries experience.
2. High esthetic requirement.
3. Bulbous teeth that are unsuitable for three-quarter crowns because it does not leave unsupported enamel.
4. Change of anterior guidance is indicated.
5. Splinting of anterior teeth.
6. The crown length is average or longer.
7. The labiolingual thickness of tooth is average or greater.

Contraindications

1. Poor oral hygiene.
2. High caries rate.
3. Young patients with large pulps.
4. Teeth that are thin labiolingually.
5. Non-vital tooth.
6. Alignment of abutment conflicts with the proposed path of withdrawal of FPD.
7. When optimum retention is required.
8. Alteration of the facial surface is required.

Advantages

1. Minimal tooth preparation.
2. Minimal margin length/gingival involvement.
3. Optimum access for margin finishing.
4. Easy to maintain hygiene.
5. Excellent esthetics.
6. Reasonable retention.

Disadvantages

1. Less retentive compared to complete coverage.
2. Technically demanding.
3. Possibility of non-vitality if the heat generated during pin preparation is not adequately managed.
4. Sometimes a slight amount of metal may be visible along the incisal edge.

RADICULAR RETAINER

- Radicular retained prosthesis consists of a post or dowel with an attached core that obtains its retention and resistance from the prepared root portion of an endodontically treated tooth.
- While the root preparation retains the post, the core establishes retention and resistance for a complete veneer crown form and functions.
  - Custom-made
  - Prefabricated

The radicular retainer is discussed in detail in the chapter on restoration of endodontically treated teeth.

RESIN-BONDED RETAINERS

- The restoration consists of one or more pontics supported by thin metal retainers placed lingual and proximally on the abutment teeth.
- These prostheses rely in part on adhesive bonding between etched enamel and metal casting.
- They are held in place by resin which locks mechanically into chemically etched enamel and also mechanically into microscopic undercuts in castings (Fig. 6.8).

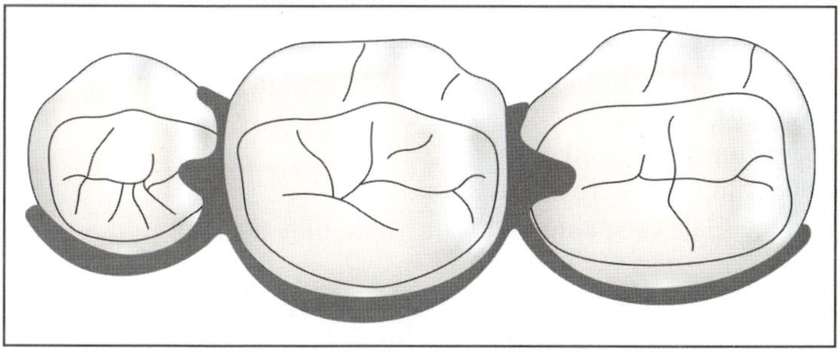

Fig. 6.8: Resin-bonded retainer replacing mandibular first molar

Indications

1. Retainers for FPD with abutments that have sufficient enamel to etch for retention, i.e. adequate crown length and bulk.
2. Splinting of periodontally compromised teeth.
3. Stabilizing dentitions after orthodontic treatment.
4. In young patients for replacements of anterior teeth.
5. In medically compromised patients.
6. Short span FPD.

7. Minimally restored or unrestored abutments.
8. Excellent moisture control possible while bonding.

Contraindications

1. Patients with parafunctional habits.
2. Long edentulous spans, replacing multiple missing teeth.
3. When facial esthetics of abutment require improvements.
4. Insufficient occlusal clearance to provide 2–3 mm vertical retention, e.g. abraded teeth.
5. Inadequate enamel surface to bond, e.g. existing restorations.
6. Incisors with extremely thin faciolingual dimensions.
7. Compromised enamel, e.g. enamel diseases.
8. Deep vertical overlap.
9. Movement of abutments that requires redistribution of pontic space.
10. High esthetic demand.
11. Nickel allergy since it is the alloy that is primarily used.[3]

Advantages

1. Conservation of tooth structure.
2. Preparation confined to enamel only, hence the potential for trauma to pulp is minimized.
3. Tissue tolerance is good because of supragingival margins.[4]
4. Anesthesia is not required since preparation is within the enamel.
5. Gingival retraction not necessary because of supragingival margins.
6. Low cost.
7. Provisional not needed.
8. Rebonding of the restorations is possible.
9. Reduced lab time since no removable dies are required.

Disadvantages

1. Longevity of prosthesis is questionable.[5]
2. Higher dislodgement rate with posterior resin retained FPD
3. Posterior metal plate may lead to graying of teeth.
4. Good abutment alignment is a must.
5. Space correction is impossible.
6. Patient should be highly motivated for adequate maintenance.
7. Over contouring is frequently encountered.

INDICATIONS FOR MULTIPLE RETAINERS

1. Abutments with short roots.
2. Lack of sufficient bone support.
3. Poor density of alveolar bone.
4. Long edentulous span.

5. Excessive lever arm action because of the shape of the anterior arch.
6. Distal extension of pontic for increased function.
7. Replacement of missing cuspid.

SELECTING THE TYPE OF RETAINER[6]

1. The amount of tooth structure of the abutment available for use—extensively decayed or restored tooth full coverage is mandatory while conservative preparations may be considered for healthy teeth.
2. The anticipated functional stress—the length of the edentulous span and dietary habits of the patient are the best indicators. Regions of high stress require full coverage.
3. The esthetic considerations—display of metal in partial coverage may limit its choice. More esthetic choice would be metal ceramic or all-ceramic retainers.
4. The laboratory facilities available—sophisticated facilities are essential for porcelain restorations.
5. The caries index and oral hygiene habits—full coverage is required in cases of high caries index and poor oral hygiene.
6. Economic considerations—patient should be able to pay for the proposed treatment.

REFERENCES

1. Lorato D.C. Effect of cervical margins on gingiva. *J Calif. Dent. Assoc* 1969; 45: 19–22.
2. Lorato DC. The effect of the crown margin extension on gingival inflammation. *J Calif. Dent. Assoc* 1969; 37: 476–8.
3. Blanco-Dalmau L. The nickel problem. *J Prosthet Dent* 1982; 48: 99.
4. Romberg, E.
5. Boening K.W. Clinical performance of resin-bonded fixed partial dentures, *J Prosthet. Dent* 1996; 76: 39–44.
6. Brehm T.W. Diagnosis and treatment planning for fixed prosthodontics, *J Prosthet. Dent* 1973; 30: 876–81.

7 Connectors

Connectors are those parts of a fixed partial denture or splint that join the individual retainers and pontics together.

CLASSIFICATION

Based on the rigidity, connectors are classified into:

A. Rigid Connectors

a. Cast
b. Soldered
c. Porcelain

B. Non-rigid Connectors

a. Key-keyway
b. Split pontic
c. Cross-pin

RIGID CONNECTORS

As the name suggests, rigid connectors form a rigid, non-movable or fixed connection between retainers and pontics or between pontics. These rigid connections can be made either by casting, soldering or welding.

Cast Rigid Connectors

These are shaped in wax connecting the wax patterns of retainers and pontics. It is a part of multiunit wax patterns, so that the bridge is cast in a single piece (Fig. 7.1).

Advantages

- Convenient.
- Minimizes the number of steps in fabrication.
- Stronger than soldered connectors.
- Easier to mask during porcelain firing.

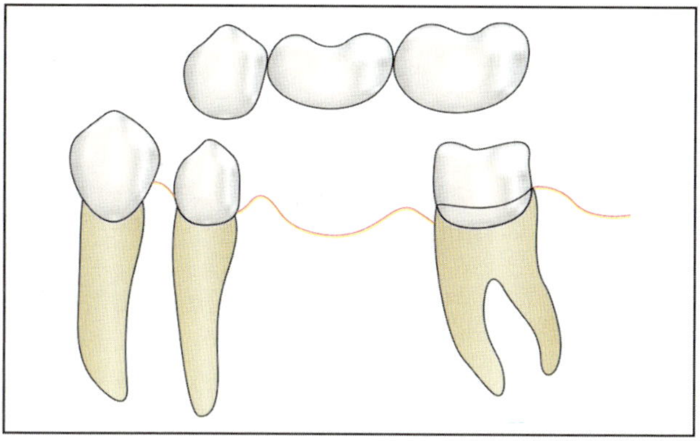

Fig. 7.1: Cast rigid connector

Disadvantages

- Makes the handling of wax patterns complex.
- Access to proximal margin is impeded and patterns cannot be held proximally during removal from the die.
- Handling of partial veneer wax pattern becomes difficult as they are easily distorted.
- Minor discrepancies in the compensation for shrinkage of metal are acceptable for single unit or small casting. However they are magnified several times in a multiple-unit casting and make it unacceptable.
- Cannot be used on distal of pier abutment.

Soldered Connectors

The retainers and pontics or portions of the fixed partial denture are cast as separate units and joined by soldering. The intermediate metal alloy usually has a lower melting temperature compared to parent metal. Although the soldering temperatures are above 450°C, the term soldering is more commonly used compared to brazing.

Similar to cast connectors, connectors to be soldered are waxed to its final shape in the wax pattern (a), a thin ribbon saw is used to cut through the wax pattern in connector area (b), the wax pattern will be cast in separate pieces. The cast pieces are assembled on the cast (c), embedded in the refractory investment material (d), and then soldered using a flame (e). Cutting a fully contoured wax pattern leaves the surfaces to be joined, flat, parallel and a controlled distance apart. The flat surfaces in the metal casting also retain heat during soldering facilitating flow of molten solder into the area. The thickness of the solder metal between the two retainers of the FPD should be evenly about 0.25 mm. Uneven thickness of the solder metal may result in distortion. Excessively thick solder impairs the strength of the prosthesis and extremely thin solder prevents proper flow of solder and a weak joint (Fig. 7.2).[1]

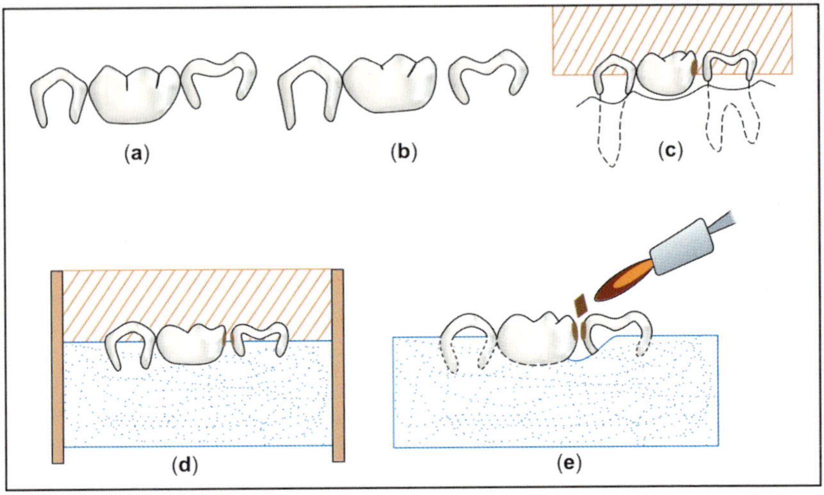

Fig. 7.2: a to e depicting the soldering procedure

Advantages

1. It simplifies the manipulation of wax patterns. The reflowing of wax along the margins, investing and casting procedures are easier.
2. Distortion of the casting is minimized as the defect is not multiplied.

Disadvantages

1. Additional steps in fabrications.
2. Dirt or surface oxides on the surface reduce wetting and impede successful soldering.
3. Accurate thickness of solder if not maintained leads to weak joint.
4. Solder metal has a different structure and usually less resistant to tarnish and corrosion.
5. The solder metal sags when subjected to higher temperature as during porcelain firing.

SOLDERING OF METAL-CERAMIC FPDS

The metal ceramic FPDs with soldered connectors may be soldered together either before or after the ceramic firing. Based on the time of soldering it is called

a. Pre-ceramic soldering
b. Post-ceramic soldering

Pre-ceramic Soldering

Once the framework is united by soldering, the subsequent steps of ceramic firing are similar to those frameworks cast in one piece. The ceramics usually have a melting temperatures less than that of the solder metal. This procedure allows the connected prosthesis to be tried in the mouth in the unglazed state. Any necessary adjustments can be made. However, contouring of the proximal surface is a little cumbersome.

Post-ceramic Soldering

The procedure is useful when the units of FPD made in different alloys are to be joined. The porcelain is fired onto the higher melting metal ceramic alloy and all adjustments including staining and glazing are completed. The unit is then joined to the other unit usually made of a regular gold alloy. The soldering is done after the proximal areas are shaped, hence the connector looks more natural than a pre-soldered or cast connector. However, any corrections required in the porcelain can be carried out only after the joint is separated.

Porcelain Connectors

They are used in conjunction with all ceramic FPDs. These connectors are formed with the more recent materials like lithium disilicate, heat pressed ceramic, empress 2 and the CAD/CAM procera systems as they have adequate strength. The connectors are part of the ceramic framework obtained by various manipulation techniques which is then layered with lower fusing porcelain. The principles of their design and position are similar to those of cast or soldered connectors. However, due to less predictability of strength, manufacturers recommend a design with larger connectors—4 × 4 mm as compared to 2 × 3 mm recommended for metal connectors. It is also recommended that an increase in the radius of curvature of the connector at the gingival area increases its resistance to fracture.[2]

Disadvantages

1. Not as strong as metal.
2. Large dimensions required.
3. Larger size leads to problems like reduced access for cleaning and impaired esthetics.

Loop Connectors

Less frequently used connectors. They are required when an existing diastema is to be maintained in a planned fixed prosthesis. The connector consists of loop of either cast metal (circular in cross section) or shaped alloy wire that connects adjacent retainers and/or pontics. This connector should be designed so that it does not interfere with functions of speech or with proper oral hygiene procedures (Fig. 7.3).

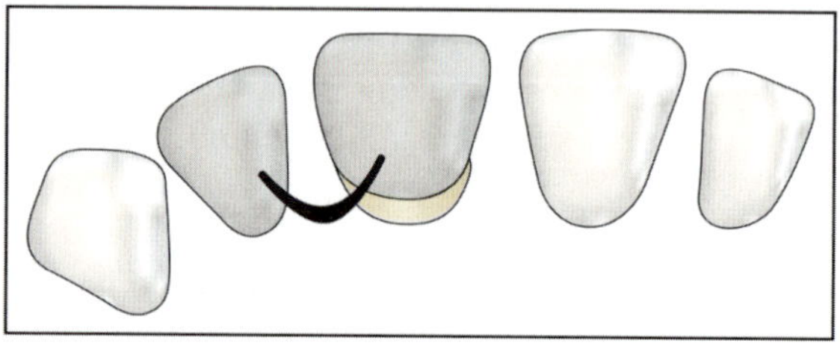

Fig. 7.3: Loop connector used to reproduce the diastema

NON-RIGID CONNECTORS

Also called movable connectors.

Indications

1. When it is not possible to prepare two abutments for an FPD with a common path of placement. The prosthesis is fabricated in two pieces and joined at the final position intraorally.
2. Doubtful prognosis of an abutment. The FPD is made in segments and if the abutment fails, only a portion of the FPD may need to be remade.
3. In large, complex FPDs where segmenting will allow easier repair and replacement of individual segments.
4. In the mandibular arch, a complex FPD consists of anterior and posterior segments. This is to allow the mediolateral flexing[3] of the mandible during opening and closing movements which would either be inhibited or to negate stresses generated that cause dislodgment of the FPD.
5. Distal surface a pier abutment. It decreases the area of maximum stress concentration.[4]

Disadvantage

Excessive tooth reduction to incorporate the connectors within the confines of the abutment.

Fabrication

During waxing of the FPD, prefabricated plastic patterns are incorporated and cast to obtain certain types of non-rigid connectors. Some others are obtained by custom milling after casting and the second part fitted to the milled retainer and then cast. Some of the commonly used non-rigid connectors are dovetails (key-keyways), split pontics (connector inside the pontic), or tapered pins.

Key-keyway

As the name suggests, the connector has a key/mortise/female component that houses the keyway/tenon/male component. The key is usually placed on the distal aspect of anterior retainers and aligned parallel to the path of withdrawal of the distal retainer. A dental surveyor may be used in aligning the components, such that when the key goes into the keyway, it should allow simultaneous placement of the second retainer into its final position. The other way is to mill a mortoise form in the pattern or casting and then fabricate the tenon part in self cure acrylic and cast separately. They are assembled in their final position in the mouth (Fig. 7.4).

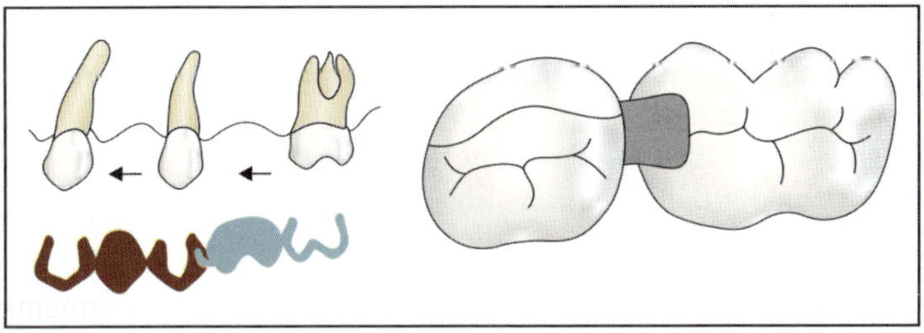

Fig. 7.4: Key and keyway connector on the distal aspect of pier abutment

Split Pontic

The attachment is placed within the pontic. The mesial half of the partial denture, i.e. mesial retainer, pontic and pier retainer are fabricated first. A distal shoe is attached to the pier retainer that represents the gingival portion of the pontic and also contains the mortise form parallel to the path of insertion of distal retainer and the tenon form in the other half of the pontic. The second part of the partial denture is fabricated separately (Fig. 7.5).

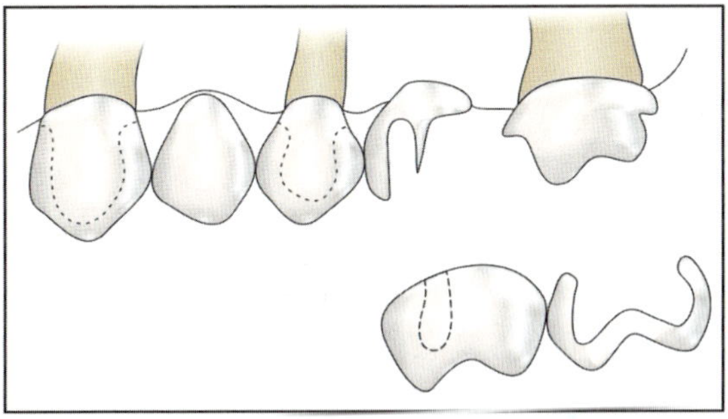

Fig. 7.5: Split pontic (maxillary first molar)

Cross Pin and Wing

This system allows the abutments to be prepared along the long axis of the tooth. A vertical wing is attached to the mesial surface of the distal retainer wax pattern. This wing should be parallel to the path of insertion of mesial abutment preparation, be 1.0 mm thick, extend 3.0 mm mesially and be short of occlusal surface by 1.0 mm. It should have a tissue surface similar to that of pontic. This is cast separately and polished. A 0.7 mm diameter hole is drilled through the wing and the casting placed on the working cast. A 0.7 mm lead is placed into the hole and the remainder of the partial denture is waxed. The lead is removed before the wax pattern is retrieved and cast separately. The two parts are assembled on the working cast. A pin is fabricated with the same metal as the casting using a pattern made from self-cure resin or by an indirect method after making an impression. The retainer with the wing is cemented first, followed by the retainer-pontic segment. The pin is seated using a punch and mallet and excess trimmed both facially and lingually. Future removal is possible by first tapping the pin out.

Pulp size and clinical crown height should be considered while designing a non-rigid connection (Fig. 7.6).

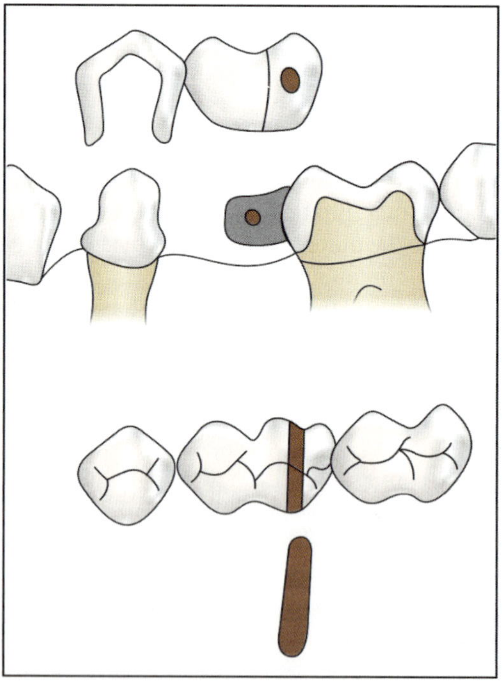

Fig. 7.6: Cross pin and wing

DESIGNING OF CONNECTORS

Connectors should have a proper size, shape and position for the success of the prosthesis. They must not fracture or distort when subjected to functional stresses. Hence they should be large. But excessively large connectors hamper oral hygiene. So the designing of connectors should be a balance between strength, esthetics and hygiene.

Strength

The connectors should be large enough without encroaching on the embrasure space. Most connectors are elliptical in shape. Such an elliptical connector is strongest if its major axis is parallel to the direction of applied force. This must be achieved whenever the esthetic and hygiene considerations permit. A minimum size of 3 × 2 mm is advisable for metal connectors, while the all-ceramic connectors require a minimum of 4 × 4 mm size (Fig. 7.7).

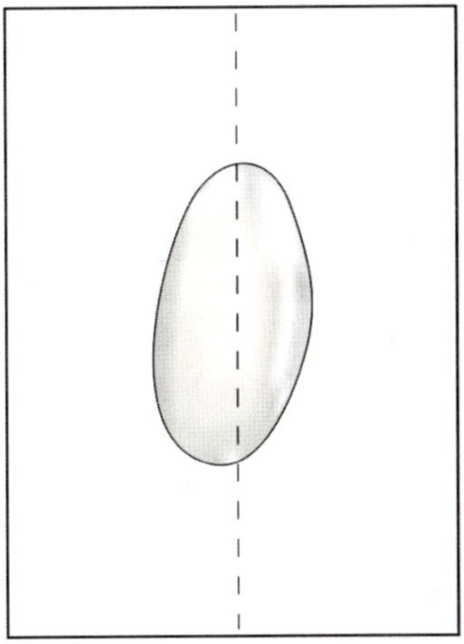

Fig. 7.7: Elliptical cross-section of connector

Esthetics

A large connector or display of metal connector due to inappropriate shaping of retainer compromises the esthetics of a restoration. For ease of cleansing, the connectors should occupy the place of interproximal contacts in the natural dentition. However, to improve appearance, in anterior FPDs connectors are placed slightly toward lingual. This position helps better shaping of retainers and does not compromise oral hygiene significantly. Mesiodistally the connector is shaped to create a smooth transition from retainer to pontic or between pontics (Fig. 7.8).

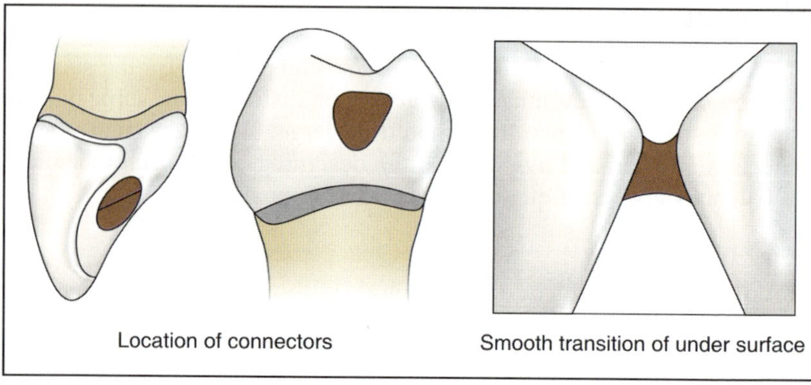

Fig. 7.8: Connectors

Hygiene

The connectors should be as small as mechanics permit. They should leave the gingival embrasures large enough to be accessed by oral hygiene aids. The under surface of the connector should be highly polished to impede plaque and calculus formation and facilitate easy cleansing. The tissue surface should be convex faciolingually to permit easy cleaning.

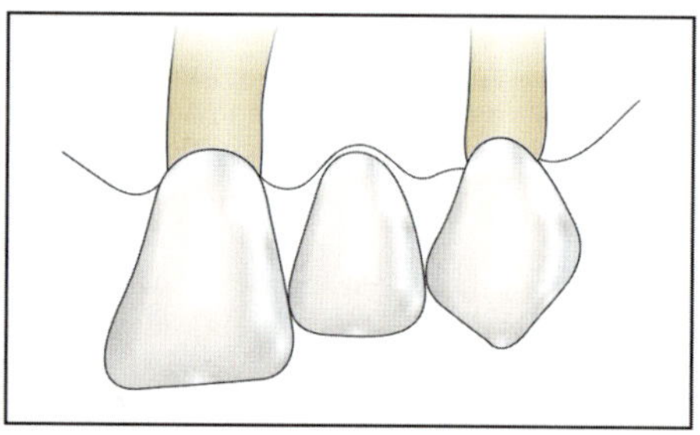

Fig. 7.9: Large gingival embrasures

REFERENCES

1. Willis L.M., Nicholls J.I. Distortion in dental soldering as affected by gap distance, *J Prosthet. Dent* 1980; 43: 272–8.
2. Won-suck O.H., Anusavice K.J. Effect of connector design on fracture resistance of all-ceramic fixed partial dentures, *J Prosthet. Dent* 2002; 87: 536–42.
3. Goodkind R.J., Heringlake C.B. Mandibular flexure in opening and closing movements. *J Prosthet. Dent* 1973; 30: 134–8.
4. Oruc S., Eraslan O., Tukay H.A., Atay A. Stress analysis of effects of nonrigid connectors on fixed partial dentures with peir abutments, *J Prosthet. Dent* 2008; 99: 185–92.

8

Pontics

GPT

1. An artificial tooth on a fixed partial denture that replaces a missing natural tooth, restores its function and usually fills the space previously occupied by the clinical crown.
2. Pontic is the suspended member of a fixed partial denture.

REQUIREMENTS

1. Pontics should restore function of mastication and speech:
   - Provide hard surface for food to be chewed
   - Restrict air passage through the edentulous area.
2. Improve appearance—fill empty spaces and provide support for lips and cheek.
3. Should provide for comfort.
4. Should be easily cleansable.
5. Be biologically acceptable.
6. Preserve the underlying mucosa.
7. Should have adequate strength.
8. Maintain the tooth relationship.

CLASSIFICATION

I. Based on Mucosal Contact

1. With mucosal contact/anatomic
   a. Ridge lap
   b. Modified ridge lap
   c. Ovate
   d. Conical
2. Non-mucosal contact/hygienic pontic
   a. Sanitary
   b. Modified sanitary or perel pontic

II. Based on Material used

1. Metal only
2. Metal ceramic
3. Combination of metal and resins

III. Based on Manufacturing

1. Custom made
2. Pre-fabricated pontics

DESIGNING PONTICS

Pontics have six surfaces

1. Gingival
2. Mesial and distal proximal
3. Occlusal
4. Buccal
5. Lingual/palatal

   Designing of each of the surfaces is considered individually.

GINGIVAL SURFACE

The various considerations which designing the gingival surface are:

1. The material
2. The shape of the surface contacting the tissue
3. Degree of tissue contact
4. Finish of the material.

Material

Various materials are available for use. Choice of material is based on esthetics and hygiene requirements. It should be non-irritating to the tissues. History or allergy to any material should be elicited before a final decision for the material is made.

Pontics should have adequate strength to resist fractures when in use. Fractures in pontics have been attributed to improper choice of materials, poor framework design, poor tooth preparation or poor occlusion. All these factors need to be taken care of while designing pontics.

Finish

Rough surfaces accumulate plaque and cause irritation. Hence, the finish of the material is more important compared to the material itself.[1] Highly glazed porcelain and finished metal surface have better biological acceptability. Compared to porous acrylic surface, their smooth surface is less retentive of plaque and easier to clean.

Contact

A pressure free contact between pontic and the underlying keratinized mucosa is desirable to prevent ulceration.[1] It is thought of as having saliva contact rather than tissue contact.[2] Necessary adjustments are made at try in using a pressure indicating paste. Pressure free contact also allows passage of oral hygiene aids.

Shape

The shape of the gingival surface is one for esthetics and another for hygiene. Therefore the location of the tooth in the mouth determines the shape of the contacting surface. In the mandibular posterior region, esthetics is not a major consideration and a spherical pontic is the design of choice. In the maxilla, the modified ridge lap design satisfies esthetics as well as hygiene. The spheroid pontic usually contacts the ridge without pressure, either on the tip of the ridge or the buccal surface. The modified ridge lap pontic contacts the labial or buccal surface without pressure in turn compensating for the loss of bone following the loss of teeth.

The sanitary pontics do not make any contact with the ridge. A minimum of 3 mm space should be given between its gingival surface and ridge. Less space causes food entrapment and sometimes tissue proliferation. The practice of scraping the cast to give tight contact between pontic and tissue is outdated. It causes inflammation and proliferation of tissues in the region. The ridge lap pontics are least recommended as they create a non-cleansable concave surface.

OCCLUSAL SURFACE

- The occlusal surface contacts the opposing dentition and provides a vertical stop.
- The positioning of the cusps is largely dictated by opposing dentition, i.e. functional cusps are to be housed in opposing fossae. The maxillary, buccal cusps are important for esthetics and to prevent cheek biting and mandibular lingual cusps prevent tongue biting. Hence their positions should not be altered.
- The reduction of the buccolingual dimension of the pontic by up to 30% is suggested to reduce forces exerted on the abutment teeth. However, this would not diminish the effects as the occlusal forces are controlled by proprioceptive mechanism and not by the size of the table.[2] In spite of that, the practice continues. The reduction in occlusal table does not reduce the forces generated during parafunctional activities when more loading is encountered. Narrowing the occlusal table is recommended in cases where the buccolingual width of the ridge is reduced, so as to facilitate plaque control measures.

PROXIMAL SURFACE

- The proximal surface must be designed to permit physiologic contours for adequate health and esthetics.
- In the maxillary anterior region, the interproximal embrasures are minimal for esthetics but should allow sufficient space to prevent papillary impingement. Posteriorly, esthetics is less critical and large embrasures are created to improve hygiene.
- Contact areas in the pontics are the location of connectors. The design of this region is discussed in the chapter on connectors.

BUCCAL AND LINGUAL SURFACE

- Esthetics, functional and hygienic requirements determine the buccal and lingual surface contours.
- In the maxilla, due to high esthetic demand the contour of facial surface, length and axial alignment cannot be altered. The lingual surface is made to harmonize with contours of adjacent teeth from cusp tip to the height of contour, and then sharply recede to the facial or buccal tissue contact area. Lingual embrasures are made larger than facial embrasures to improve access to the oral hygiene aids.
- In the mandibular posterior area, the buccal and lingual surfaces follow normal tooth form cusp tip to the height of contour and then taper towards gingival tissue contact.

PONTIC SPACE PREPARATION AND MANAGEMENT

The boundaries of pontic space are

i. Residual ridge
ii. Opposing occlusion
iii. Proximal surface of adjacent teeth
iv. Musculature of the tongue and cheek or lips. Changes in these affect the success of the restoration.

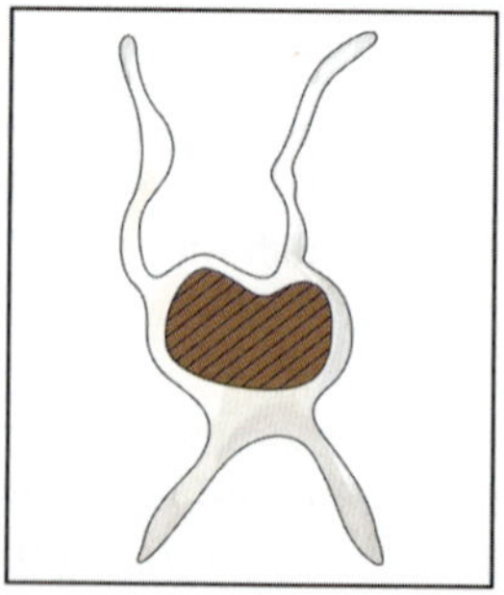

Fig. 8.1: Pontic space depicted in black colour

- The irregularities of the **residual ridge** should be corrected using surgery before the fabrication of a restoration. When the vertical height is insufficient, the ridge may be lowered and reshaped to allow for space. When an ovate/conical pontic is planned, the residual ridge is prepared by placing the gingival surface of a temporary pontic into an extraction socket/surgically prepared socket.

  The idea is to create a smooth regular surface of attached gingiva that allows maintenance of a plaque free environment. A detailed discussion of the surgical procedures involved is beyond the scope of this book.
- If the **opposing teeth** have supraerupted, occlusal plane modification is done. Based on extent, the correction may require single surface grinding to intentional RCT and crown. The procedure should be carried out before construction of FPD.
- If **adjacent teeth** have migrated into edentulous space, orthodontics may be indicated to improve pontic contour, periodontal health and to ensure transmission of forces along the axis of abutment. Mild migrations may, however, be managed during abutment preparation. Diagnostic waxing will help determine the amount of alteration required in the preparation.
- The pontic should be positioned away from **movable mucosa** to prevent tissue proliferation around the pontic. The surface should not irritate the tongue and cheek mucosa.
- **Increased ridge resorption** may leave a longer pontic when pontic is designed to simulate natural tooth contours. Such a situation is managed either by ridge augmentation or by modification of pontic design. The gingival half of the labial surface may be recontoured to produce the illusion of normal length. In excessive resorption, pontic may be shaped as crown and root with staining to simulate exposed dentin or gingival tissues.

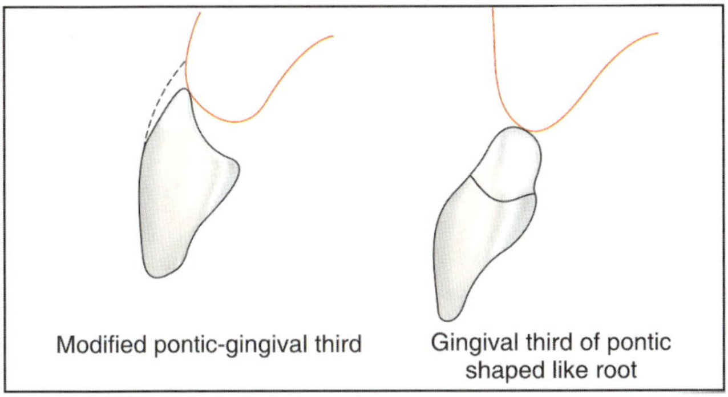

Fig. 8.2

- Uncontrolled teeth movement may cause an increase in **mesiodistal width** of pontic space. Severe cases may require orthodontic correction. However in milder cases, the illusion of normal width pontic can be created by keeping the positions of mesiofacial and distofacial line angles similar to contralateral tooth and altering the shape of proximal areas. A space discrepancy in posterior can be managed by keeping mesial half similar while adjusting the size of the distal half [Fig. 8.3(a to c)].

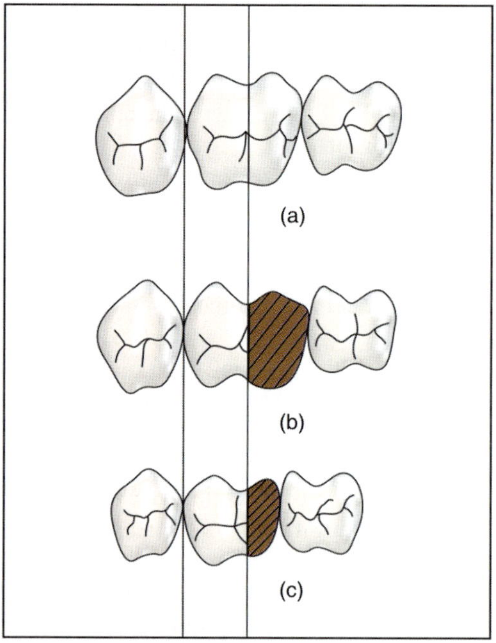

Fig. 8.3

In multi-pontic situations it may be best to eliminate interpontic gingival embrasures.[3] This enhances hygiene as well as adds strength to the pontic. This may limit or eliminate soft tissue proliferation.[4]

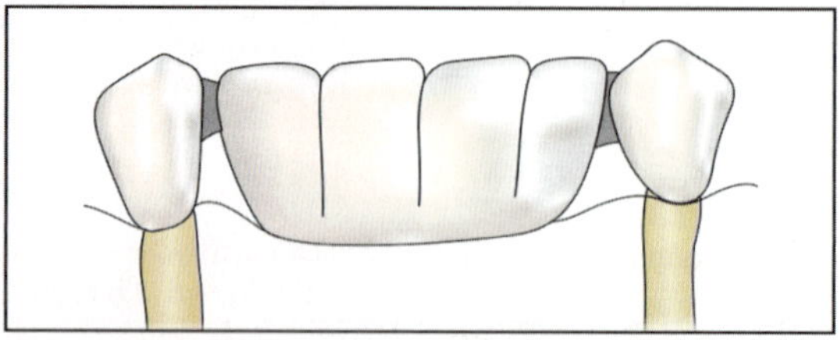

Fig. 8.4: Fused pontics

Information box: Seibert's[5] classification for residual ridge deformities:

Class I defects	Faciolingual loss of tissue width with normal ridge height.
Class II defects	Loss of ridge height with normal ridge width.
Class III defects	A combination of loss in both dimensions.

DISCUSSION OF PONTICS

1. Ridge Lap Pontic or Saddle Pontic

The saddle pontic overlaps the residual ridge buccolingually, simulating the contours and emergence profile of the missing tooth on both sides of the residual ridge (Fig. 8.5).

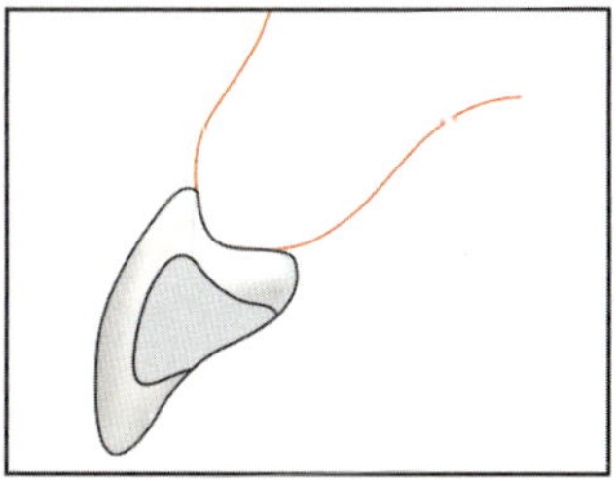

Fig. 8.5: Saddle pontic

Advantage

Good esthetics

Disadvantage

The concave gingival surface of the pontic is not accessible to cleaning with the dental floss, which will lead to plaque accumulation and result in tissue inflammation.

2. Modified Ridge Lap Pontic

- Stein's article on pontic design lead to the popularization of this design.[6]
- Combines the best features of the hygienic and saddle pontic designs; esthetics with easy cleansing.
- It overlaps the residual ridge on the facial but remains clear of the ridge on the lingual.
- To enable optimal plaque control, the gingival surface must have no depression or hollow; rather, it must be as convex as possible from mesial to distal.
- Tissue contact should resemble the letter T whose vertical arm ends at the crest of the ridge.

- Facial ridge adaptation is essential for a natural appearance.
- The adaptation should be such that no shadow is cast in the gingival area. The result would be unesthetic.
- The modified ridge lap design is the most common pontic form used in areas of the mouth that are visible during function (Fig. 8.6).

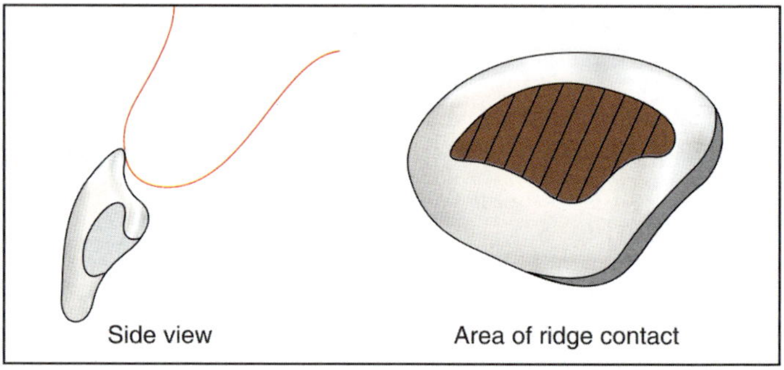

Fig. 8.6: Modified ridge lap pontic

3. Conical Pontic = Egg Shaped/Bullet Shaped/Heart Shaped Pontic

- It should be made as convex as possible, with only one point of contact at the center of the residual ridge or slightly buccal.
- This design is recommended for the replacement of mandibular posterior teeth where esthetics is a lesser concern.
- The facial and lingual contours are dependent on the width of the residual ridge; a knife-edged residual ridge will necessitate flatter contours with a narrow tissue contact area.
- This type of design may be unsuitable for broad residual ridges, because the emergence profile associated with the small tissue contact point may create areas of food entrapment.

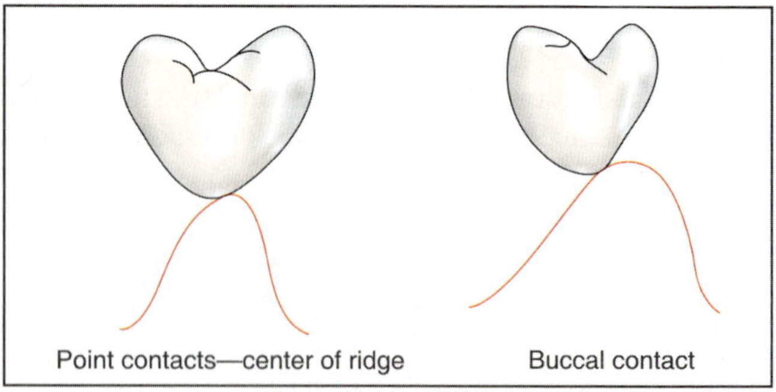

Fig. 8.7: Conical pontic

4. Ovate Pontic

- The ovate pontic is the most esthetically appealing pontic design.
- Its convex tissue surface resides in a soft tissue depression or a hollow in the residual ridge, which makes it appear that a tooth is literally emerging from the gingiva.
- Careful treatment planning is necessary for successful results.
- Socket preservation techniques should be performed at the time of extraction to create tissue recess from which the ovate pontic form will emerge.
- For a pre-existing residual ridge, soft tissue surgical augmentation is typically required. When an adequate volume of ridge tissue is established, a socket depression is sculpted into the ridge with surgical diamonds or electrosurgery.
- In either case, meticulous attention to the contour of the pontic of the provisional restoration is essential when conditioning and shaping the residual ridge that will receive the definitive prosthesis.

Advantages

1. Pleasing appearance
2. Strength—the broad convex geometry is stronger than that of the ridge lap pontic, because the unsupported, thin porcelain that often exists at the gingivofacial extent is eliminated.
3. Recessed form—not susceptible to food impaction.
4. Convex in all dimensions—accessible to dental floss.

Disadvantages

1. Meticulous oral hygiene is necessary to prevent tissue inflammation from large area of tissue contact.
2. Need for surgical tissue management.
3. Need for patient co-operation
4. Cost.

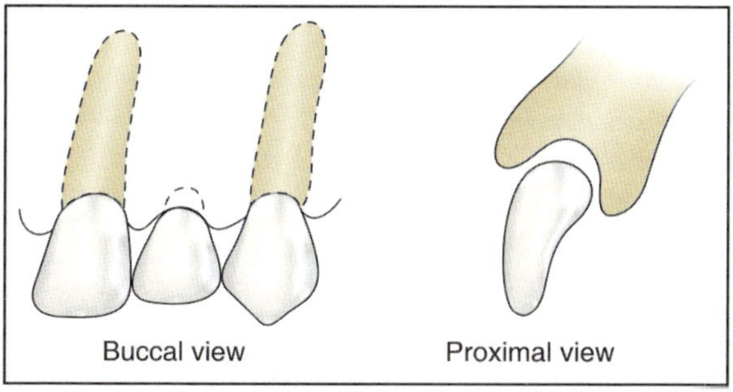

Fig. 8.8: Ovate pontic

5. Sanitary/Hygienic Pontic

- Tissue surface remains clear of the residual ridge.
- Plaque control is easy.
- Least "tooth like" design and is therefore reserved for teeth seldom displayed during function.
- *Disadvantage:* Entrapment of food particles that may lead to tongue habits that may annoy the patient.

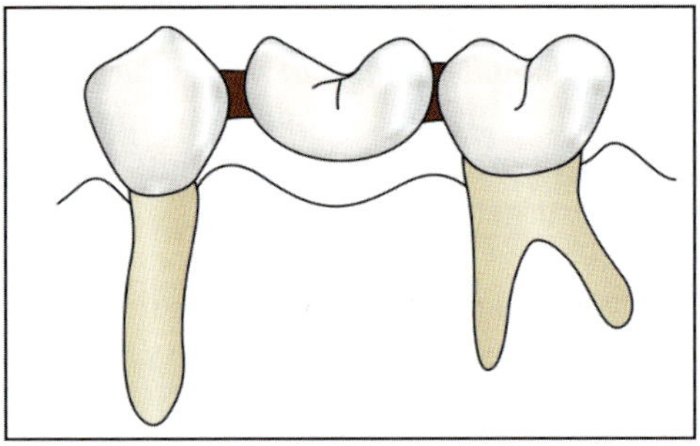

Fig. 8.9: Sanitary pontic

6. Modified Sanitary Pontic

- Gingival portion shaped like an archway between retainers.
- Geometry permits increased connector size while decreasing the stress concentrated in the pontic and connectors.
- No criteria are established for minimum thickness. Clinical judgment dictates at least the occlusal third should be used.

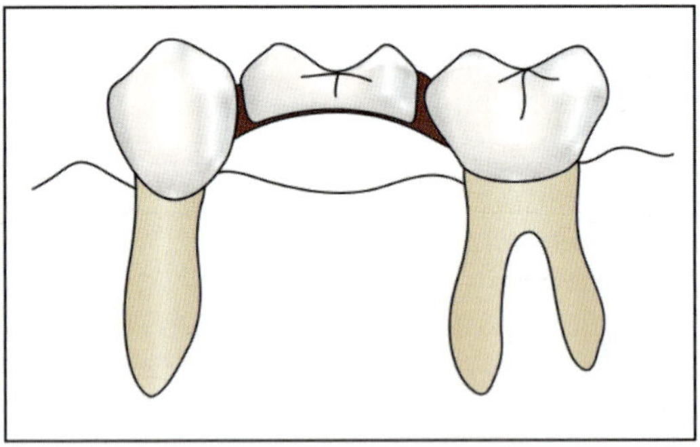

Fig. 8.10: Modified sanitary pontic

- The thickness may be increased in cases of long span FPD.
- Perel has summarized the advantages as[7]
  1. Makes food retention impossible

2. Easy to clean
3. Prevents flexure of prosthesis
4. Reshapes and reinforces the critical solder joint
5. Less susceptible to tissue proliferation.

7. Prefabricated Pontics[8]

a. The Flatback Facing

- Nearest to being interchangeable.
- Has incisal path of insertion.
- Positioned slightly short of occlusal plane to protect the porcelain from positive biting forces.

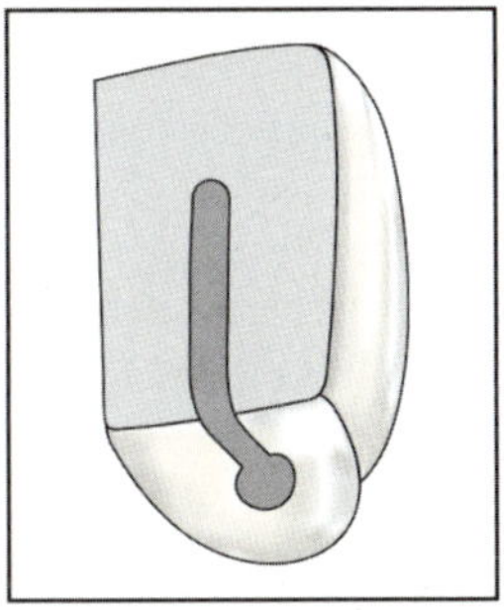

Fig. 8.11: Prefabricated pontic—the flatback facing

b. The Truspontic Facings

- Do not select on interchangeability
  i. Additional strength is attained in the backing when the occlusal edge is beveled and lingual slope is hollow ground.
  ii. Normal width and plenty of occlusogingival space is needed to use the facing successfully.
  iii. Acceptable for maxillary posteriors

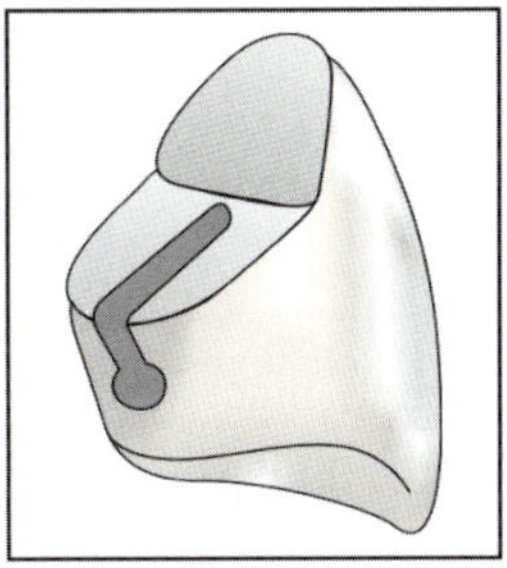

Fig. 8.12: Prefabricated pontic—the truspontic facings

c. The Long Pin Facings

- Adapted to largest number of situations.
  - i. In areas of short vertical height.
  - ii. Medium fusing porcelain may be added to tissue surface.
  - iii. Contraindicated if opposing teeth have a large vertical overlap.
  - iv. Space width must be greater than that between the retention pins.

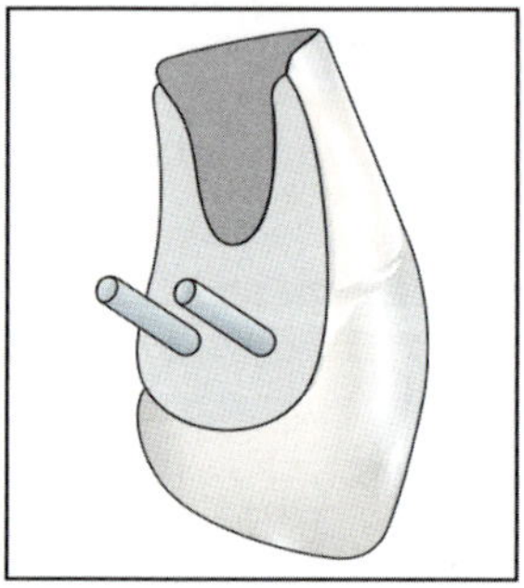

Fig. 8.13: Prefabricated pontic—the long pin facings

d. The Reverse Pin Facing

- Fabricated from porcelain denture tooth using a special porcelain drill press.
- Excellent esthetics can be attained in the anterior part of mouth.
- Retention is secured over the entire lingual surface.

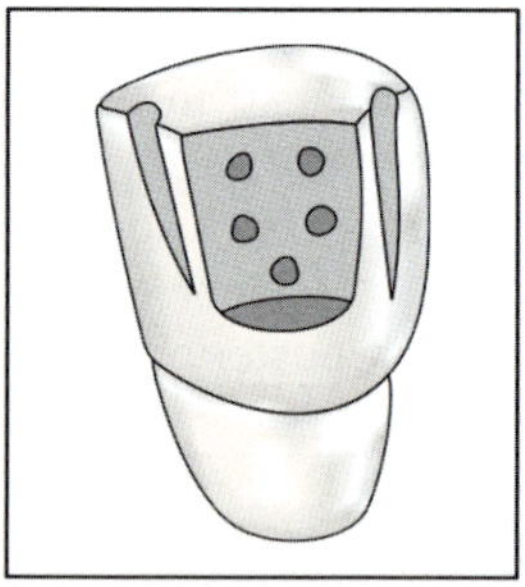

Fig. 8.14: Prefabricated pontic—the reverse pin facing

e. The Sanitary Facings

- Provides porcelain on ridge contact surface.
- Not indicated when the edentulous space is extremely narrow in width and length.
- Used exclusively in the lower dental arch.

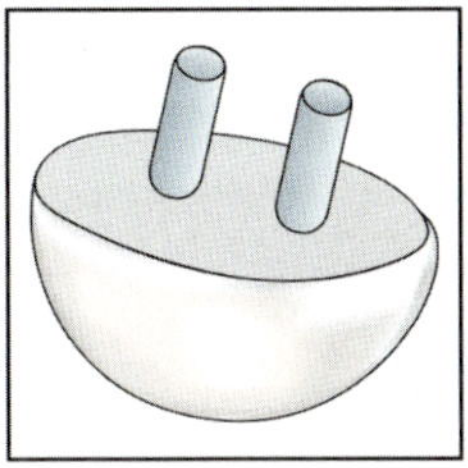

Fig. 8.15: Prefabricated pontic—the sanitary facings

8. Fused Pontics

When the edentulous span is long, as in case of missing lower incisors being replaced by an FPD, the gingival embrasure spaces are merged together. This minimizes food retention in the area and increases the strength of the pontics.

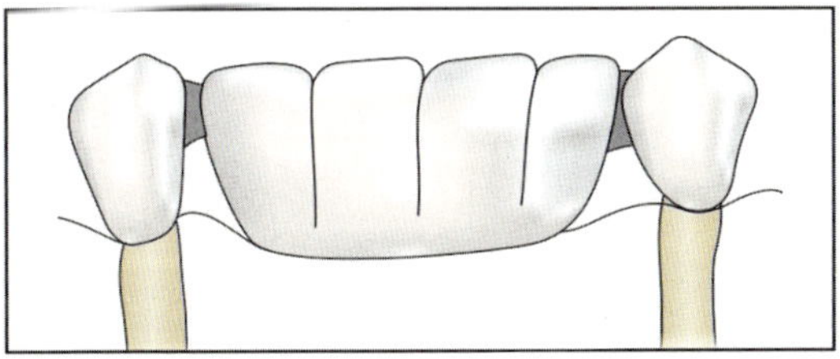

Fig. 8.16: Fused pontics

REFERENCES

1. Cavazos E. Tissue response to fixed partial denture pontics, *J Prosthet. Dent* 1968; 2: 143–53.
2. Reynolds J.M. Abutment selection for fixed prosthodontics. *J Prosthet. Dent* 1968; 19: 483–8.
3. Porter P.D. Jr., Anterior pontic design: a logical progression. *J Prosthet. Dent* 1986; 51:774–6.
4. Crispin B.J. Tissue response to posterior denture base type pontics. *J Prosthet. Dent* 1979; 42: 257–61.
5. Siebert J.S. Reconstruction of deformed, partially edentulous ridge, using full thickness onlay grafts. Part I. Technique and wound healing. *Compend Contin. educ. Dent* 1983; 4: 437–53.
6. Stein R.S. Pontic-residual ridge relationship. A research report. *J Prosthet. Dent* 1966; 16: 251–85.
7. Perel M.L. A modified sanitary pontic. *J Prosthet. Dent* 1972; 28: 589–92.
8. Reynolds M.J. Selecting facings for pontics. *J Prosthet. Dent* 1964;14: 746–51.

PART III
Clinical Procedures

9

Shade Selection

Matching the shade or color of a restoration to that of the adjacent natural teeth is an important aspect of the practice of fixed prosthodontics. Success or failure of a restoration may entirely depend on this aspect. Culpepper pointed out the inconsistencies among dentists to match the natural tooth shades and their inability to duplicate their selections from one time to another.[1] Dr. E. Bruce Clark was the first to describe the proper use of color in the dental profession. A brief introduction to color is essential before shade selection may be understood.

COLOR

Color is a phenomenon of light or visual perception that permits differentiation of otherwise identical objects. When light falls on an object, it is modified by being partly absorbed, reflected, refracted or transmitted by the object. When this light enters the human eye, it is perceived as a particular color. Thus, color is influenced by:

1. Physical properties of the object
2. Nature of the incident light
3. Surrounding colored objects
4. The subjective analysis of the observer
5. Angle of observation
6. Light and dark adaptation
7. Size of the field of view

MUNSELL COLOR ORDER SYSTEM

It is the most popular method for describing color. It describes color as an entity with three dimensions, viz. hue, value and chroma. It is possible to vary each of these qualities without disturbing the other.

Hue

In Munsell's words "it is that quality by which we distinguish one color family from another, as red from yellow, green from blue or purple." It is determined by the wavelength of the reflected or transmitted light that is observed. In the Munsell color system, hue is divided into 10 gradations—yellow (Y), yellow–red (YR), red (R), red–purple (RP), purple (P), purple–blue (PB), blue (B), blue–green (BG), green (G) and green–yellow (GY). Each gradation is subdivided, e.g. 1 R, 2R–10R, which in turn is subdivided into 1.1R, 1.2R–2R. So, a hue may be represented as 3.2 Y or 7.1 GY. The hues of most natural teeth fall between yellow and yellow–red.

Chroma

Chroma "is that quality by which we distinguish a strong color from a weak one; the departure of a color sensation from that of white or gray." It defines the saturation or intensity of a hue. The chroma measurements start from zero, or achromatic, with increasing numbers indicating stronger colors. The maximum chroma depends on a particular hue but can range from 10 to 14. Natural teeth may have a chroma from 0.5 to 4.

Value

Value "is that quality by which we distinguish a light color from a dark color." Or simply, value of a color is the gray it would match if it were seen on a black and white television screen. It is a direct consequence of the amount of light the color reflects or transmits. The possible range of values in Munsell color system is from zero for black to 10 for white. Natural teeth have a value between 5.5 and 8.5. Value is considered the most important of the three dimensions because a restoration with very high brightness is easily detectable even to an untrained eye.

Advantages of Munsell color order system:[2]

1. Consistency
2. Flexibility
3. Simplicity
4. Worldwide recognition
5. Attempt to achieve equal visual (perceptual) spacing in the system
6. Hues projecting unevenly beyond the surface of the solid allows the addition of purer colors to the periphery as and when technology permits their creation.

CIELAB COLOR SYSTEM

The CIELAB color system was determined by the commission internationale de l'eclairage in 1978. 'L' is the equivalent of value, whereas 'a' and 'b' denote the chromatic characteristics of the color. The CIELAB color system is gaining acceptance in dental research. Using certain numerical parameters, the CIELAB measurements can be correlated to the hue, chroma and value measurements of the Munsell system.

GUIDELINES FOR CLINICAL SHADE SELECTION

1. Lighting

- The standard daylight or the Northern exposure sunlight in the middle portion of a day is considered the optimal source.
- Color-corrected fluorescent lighting is recommended in daily practice because it approaches the necessary type of balance.
- The recommended amount of lighting is about three ceiling fixtures, each containing four 48 inch tubes installed in a 10 feet by 10 feet room.
- Brightly colored surrounding objects may change the nature of light reaching the patients. A light gray is the ideal background. Lipstick and heavy makeup should be removed before shade selection.

2. Patient Position

- The patient should be seated upright and at the observer's eye level.

3. Tooth Condition

- The teeth should be polished to remove plaque and stains.
- Teeth should be moist. Dry teeth have higher value.

4. Distance

- Selection should be made at 3 to 6 feet from the oral cavity to simulate the conditions under which the restoration will most commonly be observed.
- Also, it helps in easier selection of value.

SEQUENCE OF SHADE SELECTION

- It is preferable to use the same shade guide the manufacture used in designating the colors of the product.
- Eliminate the tabs that are the worst match.
- When the necks of the tabs exhibit excessive colorants, remove them to minimize distraction.
- It is important to match the shade before preparation of teeth is initiated
- First, the nearest hue is chosen, followed by matching the chroma and value.
- *Hue selection:* In a typical shade guide (vita lumin), the hue have been grouped into A1, A2, A3, A3.5 and A4 and so are B, C and D shades. The region with the highest chrome, i.e. cervical region of canines is used for initial hue selection.
- *Chroma selection:* Once the hue is selected, the best match within the available gradations for chroma is matched.
- *Value selection:* A separate value-ordered shade guide is used to check lightness. The selection is best done by observing from a distance and

squinting the eyes. Squinting helps by increasing sensitivity to achromatic conditions. The observer should concentrate on which disappears from the sight first—the tooth or the shade tab. The one that fades first has the lower value. Now, the selected value is compared to the value of the selected hue and chroma. If the value selected is lower, a repeat of hue and chroma selection is usually necessary.

PROBLEMS DURING SHADE SELECTION

1. Color Adaptation[3]

The cones present in the retina sense color and are fatigued very fast. On continuous observation, the color vision decreases, whereas the chroma of complementary colors appears greater. Thus, painting the operatory pale blue or glancing at a gray-blue surface periodically can help in color selection.

2. Metamerism

Two colors that match under a given lighting but have different spectral reflectance are called metamers, and the phenomenon is called metamerism. For example, an object may appear yellow when actually it reflects orange and green light in particular lighting condition. When the lighting condition is changed, the color no longer matches. The problem can be minimized by selecting a shade and confirming it under different lighting conditions.

3. Fluorescence

Some objects absorb radiant energy and re-emit the energy at a lower frequency than it is absorbed. Such objects are known to be florescent. Tooth enamel is florescent. A mismatch can occur if the dental restoration has different florescence than enamel. This phenomenon, however, does not play a very significant role in color matching.[4]

4. Color Blindness

About 8% of the male population has defects in color vision. The incidence is lesser in female population. Different types of color blindness exist, from complete lack of color sensitivity to lack of one primary color vision. The dentist should get his color vision examined and should seek assistance when selecting the shade.[5]

5. Surrounding Colors

Light strikes a variety of objects in the operatory before it falls on the tooth. Thus, even a light from a good source may be modified and rendered unacceptable. The dentist's or patient's brightly colored clothes can reflect undesirable colors. A drape may be used to mask this. Lipstick should be removed before color selection. A color-corrected light may be used for oral lighting. A proper (light gray) background may be used for color matching.

REQUIREMENTS OF A SHADE GUIDE[6]

1. A logical arrangement in color space.
2. An adequate distribution in color space.

Such a shade guide helps fasten the procedure and also helps to check logically the chosen match for accuracy.

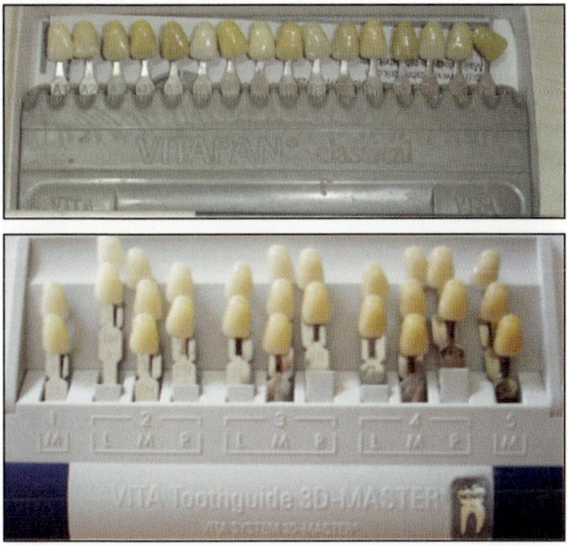

Fig. 9.1: Vitapan 2D and 3D shade guides—commonly used in shade selection

3D Master

1. The values of all shades are grouped into 5 groups.
2. The different chroma levels are grouped in the vertical axis.
3. The hue values are depicted in the horizontal axis—yellowish hue to the left and reddish hue to the right of the group (L–R).

REFERENCES

1. Culpepper W.D. A comparative study of shade-matching procedures. *J Prosthet. Dent* 1970; 24: 166–73.

2. Sproull R.C. Color matching in dentistry, Part I. The three-dimensional nature of color. *J Prosthet. Dent* 1973; 20: 416–24.
3. Cohen J. Color adaptation of the human eye, *Am. J. Psychology* 1946; 59: 84–110.
4. Seghi R.R., Johnston W.M. Estimate of colorimetric measurement errors associated with natural tooth fluorescence, *J Dent. Res* 1992; 71:303 (Abstract no. 1578).
5. Davison S.P., Myslinski N.R. Shade selection by color vision defective dental personnel, *J Prosthet. Dent* 1990; 63: 97–101.
6. Sproull R.C. Color matching in dentistry, Part II. Practical applications of the organization of color. *J Prosthet. Dent* 1973; 29: 556–66.

10

Principles of Tooth Preparation

Tooth preparation is defined as the mechanical treatment of dental disease or injury to hard tissues that restores a tooth to the original form.

Once the diagnosis is made, a treatment plan is determined. Based on the determined treatment plan, a series of procedures are to be carried out. When it is decided to place an FPD to replace the missing teeth, the selected abutment teeth are to be prepared to receive the retainers. A set of guidelines are to be followed while preparation so that the restoration is biologically, mechanically and esthetically acceptable within the oral environment. These guidelines are called the principles of tooth preparation and aptly grouped by Rosensteil[1] into:

I. Biologic considerations
II. Mechanical considerations
III. Esthetic considerations.

A successful restoration requires simultaneous consideration of all these factors. A skilled clinician is one who finds the best combination of compromises among all these principles.

BIOLOGIC CONSIDERATIONS

The measures taken to prevent any damage to the existing tissues, conservation of maximum tooth structure, obtaining an occlusion that is harmonious with the existing condition and long-term protection and maintenance of tooth and restoration are the factors to be considered in this section.

a. Prevention of Damage

- *Tooth being prepared:* The teeth need to be protected against excessive heat generated due to friction while preparation. The heat may increase due to excessive pressure, higher rotational speeds, type, shape and condition of the cutting instrument.[2] The heat buildup may be reduced by the use of a coolant water spray. Chemical agents used to clean prepared tooth surfaces act as pulpal irritants[3] and should not be used.

All existing restorations should be carefully evaluated for signs of pulpal damage. If the need be, the tooth should be RCT treated to avoid jeopardy of extensive prosthetic treatment due to residual infections within the pulp.

- *Adjacent teeth:* Any damage of adjacent teeth should be avoided as this violates the surface enamel layer that is high in fluoride content and makes the surface prone to dental caries. Use of metal matrix band or a thin lip/ fin of the tooth being prepared are the preferred methods to reduce this damage (Fig. 10.1).

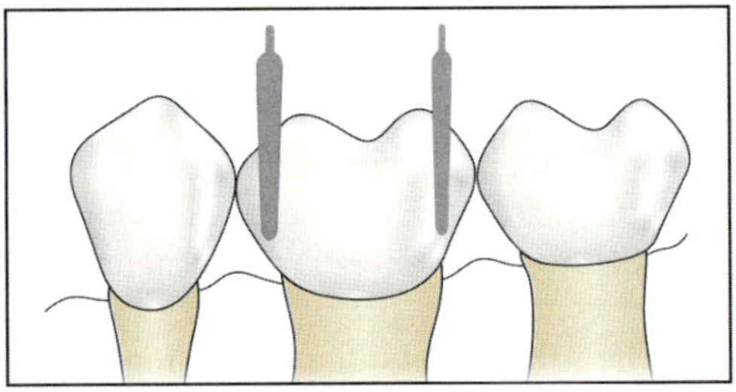

Fig. 10.1: Thin lip on either sides protect the adjacent teeth

- *Soft tissues:* The cheeks and tongue need to be adequately protected with mouth mirrors, aspirator tip and saliva ejectors. The bur should not be rotating while moving the handpiece in and out of the mouth. The gingival tissue may be protected by retraction with cords during preparation to minimize damage. This also increases access and visibility in the area.
- *Preservation of periodontium:* Proper selection of margins, adequate reduction to facilitate proper contours contribute to preserve the periodontium.
- *TMJ:* Excessive stretching and long hours of preparation may lead to damage to TMJ. Adequate care should be taken towards this fact at the diagnosis and tooth preparation stages.

b. Conservation of Tooth Structure

- *Partial coverage restorations* are conservative of tooth structure because they involve less number of surfaces and should be used whenever feasible.
- *Taper:* Preparations with minimal taper not only conserve tooth structure but also help in retention (Fig. 10.2).
- *Preservation of anatomy:* The cuspal planes should be reduced evenly to protect the anatomy as well as the pulp horns that are pointed towards the cusp. This kind of reduction also adds to the structural durability of the restorations.

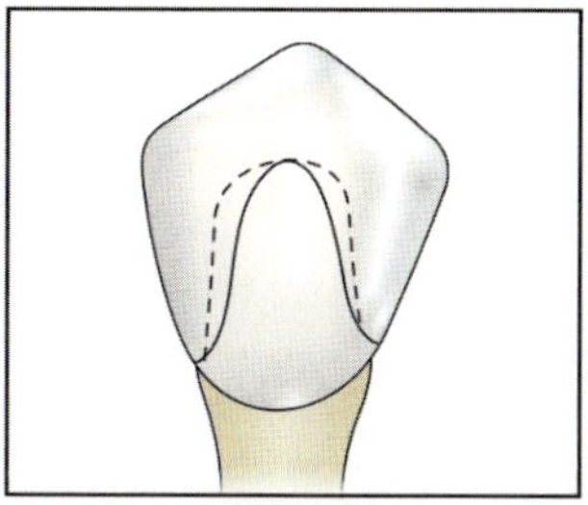

Fig. 10.2: Correct taper (dotted lines) conserves tooth structure

- *Dentin thickness:* Preserve as much of the dentin as possible as this has been shown to be inversely proportional to the pulpal response.
- *Margin selection:* In accordance with the other principles, the most conservative margin type should be selected.
- *Apical extension:* Unnecessary extension of the preparation (e.g. subgingival placement of margins) should be avoided.
- *Uprighting molars:* When the axial position or angulation of abutments is not ideal, the use of orthodontic repositioning may be considered to conserve tooth structure (Fig. 10.3).

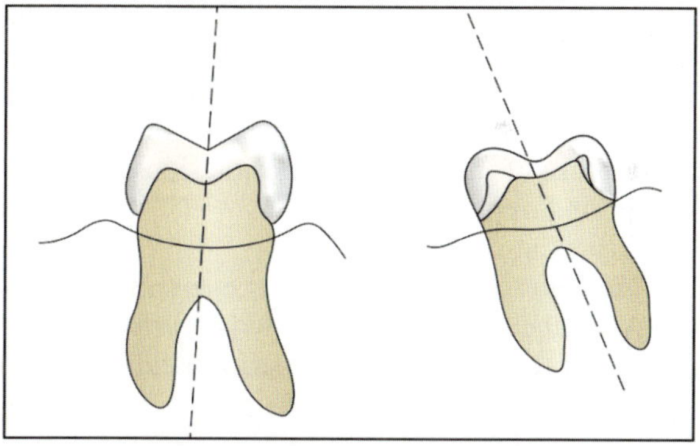

Fig. 10.3: Tilted molars need excessive reduction (darkened) to obtain parallel path of insertion

c. Considerations for Long-term Health and Success of Restoration

- *Adequate axial reduction:* It is essential to obtain correct contours of the restoration. Overcontoured restorations may lead to plaque accumulation around gingival margins,[4] dental caries or periodontal disease[5] on the long run. Correct contours are also important for adequate esthetics of the restoration.
- *Position of margins:* When factors permit, a supragingival margin should always be chosen over subgingival margins (Fig. 10.4).

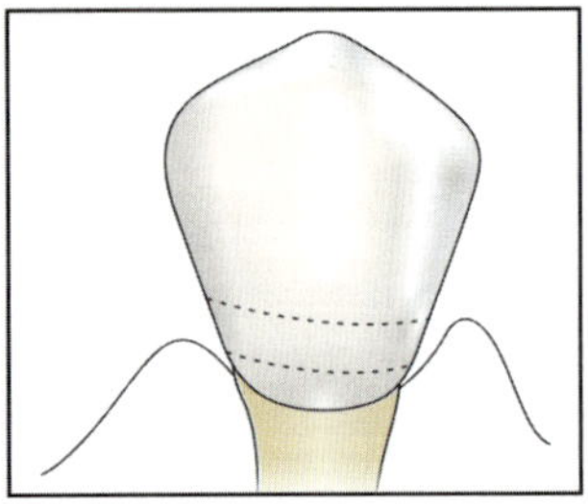

Fig. 10.4: Location of supragingival and subgingival margins

Advantages of supragingival margins

- Do not contribute to periodontal disease.[6]
- Easy to prepare and finish.
- Located on enamel.
- Do not damage soft tissues during preparation or impressions.
- Easy to record.
- Easy to maintain.
- Easy to evaluate at recall appointments.

Factors that justify the use of subgingival margins

- High caries index.
- Dental disease or previous restorations extending subgingivally.
- Essential so as to comfortably break interproximal contacts.
- Esthetics as in case of metal ceramic restorations.
- Need for additional retention.
- Need to modify axial contours.

Adaptation of margins: Smooth margins are essential to obtain a well-fitting casting. When the restoration is adapted accurately to the tooth, there are lesser chances of recurrent caries or periodontal disease (Fig. 10.5).[7]

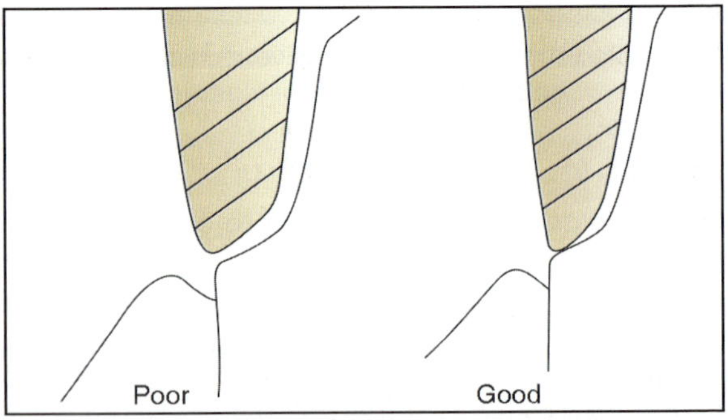

Fig. 10.5: Adaptation of margins

- *Type of margins:* A variety of margins are described.[8] The featheredge is the most conservative of tooth structure. However, its use is contraindicated in most of the cases because of its disadvantages. Various factors should be considered before the correct margin type is selected. The chamfer, heavy chamfer, shoulder and shoulder with bevel are the most commonly used margins for cast restorations.
- *Occlusion:* The final restoration should result in a harmonious occlusion. The existing occlusal plane should be carefully evaluated and the teeth reduced accordingly. When the patient's occlusal plane is disrupted by factors like supra-erupted teeth or tilted teeth, it may be necessary to violate the principle of conservation than the result being a traumatic occlusion. Diagnostic preparations on the cast and wax up may help to decide if an intentional RCT is required.
- *Protection of teeth:* All intracoronal cast restorations act as wedges trying to split the teeth. If the remaining tooth structure is insufficient to resist such a fracture, cuspal coverage should be provided. Although onlays and crowns are less conservative of tooth structure, on the long run they reduce the chances of fracture of the prepared tooth.

MECHANICAL CONSIDERATIONS

The mechanical considerations include those measures to improve the retention of the restoration, reduce its dislodgement under forces other than along the long axis (resistance), and deformation of the restoration when in function.

1. Retention Form

This is the resistance of the restoration to dislodgement under forces that are parallel to the long axis. Loss of retention is one of the most common causes of failure of FPD.

- *Dislodging forces:* The common dislodging forces are pulling by sticky foods and pressure from floss under the connector. However, the magnitude of these forces is small and the patient may be advised regarding the same.
- *Taper of the preparation:* Since cast restorations are rigid and cannot flex over undercuts, the preparations cannot have perfect parallel walls. A minimal taper limits the path of withdrawal to a single path and thus effectively increases the frictional resistance provided by the cement placed between the tooth and restoration. The recommended taper for the preparation is 6° which has been shown to optimize retention for zinc phosphate cement.[9]
- *Area of prepared axial surfaces:* Supposing the prepared tooth has minimal taper, the retention of the restoration depends on the length of

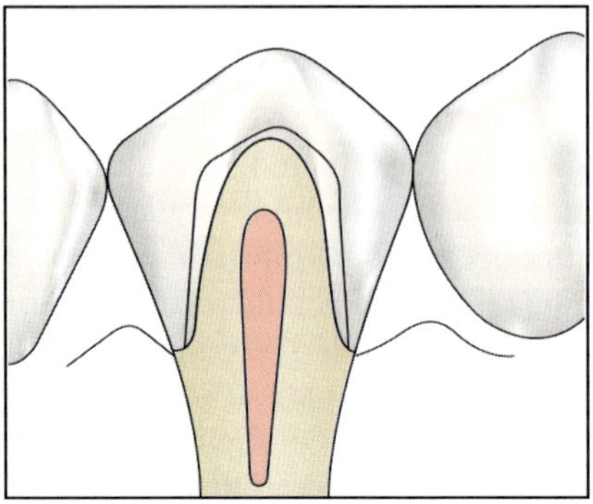

Fig. 10.6: Minimal taper-better retention

the preparation. Crowns with long axial walls have better retention than those with short ones[10] and molars have better retention than premolar crowns of the same taper. Since the restoration tends to lift off rather than slide over the occlusal surfaces, these surfaces do not contribute to retention of the restoration (Fig. 10.6).

A complete crown is more retentive than a partial crown because of its increased surface area. The addition of grooves in partial coverage crowns increases retention by limiting the path of withdrawal rather than by increasing the area.

- *Sharp line angles:* Sharp line angles within the preparation especially along the junction of axial and occlusal surfaces lead to stress concentration. This leads to a cohesive failure within the cement layer and loss of retention. The internal line angles should therefore be rounded.
- *Roughness of casting:* Retention is shown to increase when the internal surface of the restoration is roughened or grooved.[11] However, retention is not affected when the tooth surface is roughened. This is not recommended also because it complicates impression making and waxing procedures.
- *Casting alloy:* The more reactive the alloy, better the retention. Base metal alloys are better retained as compared to gold alloys.[12]
- *Luting agent:* In general, the adhesive resin cements have been shown to be the most retentive cements.[13]
- *Cement thickness:* Generally thicker the cement layer, less effective is the frictional resistance to removal. However, the studies regarding this are inconclusive.

2. Resistance Form

- Rotational forces are active within the oral cavity and the crown may act as a ring. The rotation may be resisted by any surface that is perpendicular to these forces (Fig. 10.7).

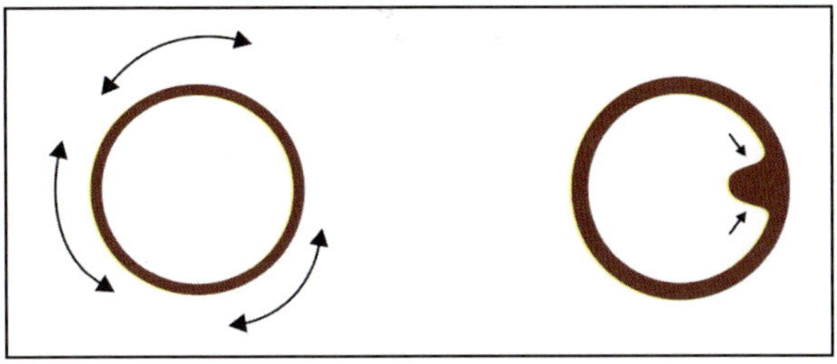

Fig. 10.7: Surfaces introduced to resist rotational forces

- This is *resistance to dislodgement* under forces other than along long axis of teeth. These forces are usually greater than those trying to dislodge the restoration along its long axis, especially in patients with parafunctional habits (Fig. 10.8).

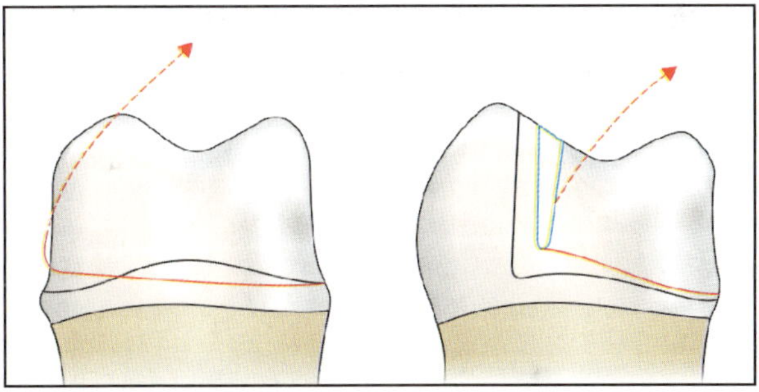

Fig. 10.8: Tipping forces tend to dislodge the restoration along the arc of rotation (red)

- *Taper:* Increase in taper decreases resistance.
- *Length of preparation:* Shorter preparations have a very little resistance, hence they require a more parallel preparation (Fig. 10.9).[14]

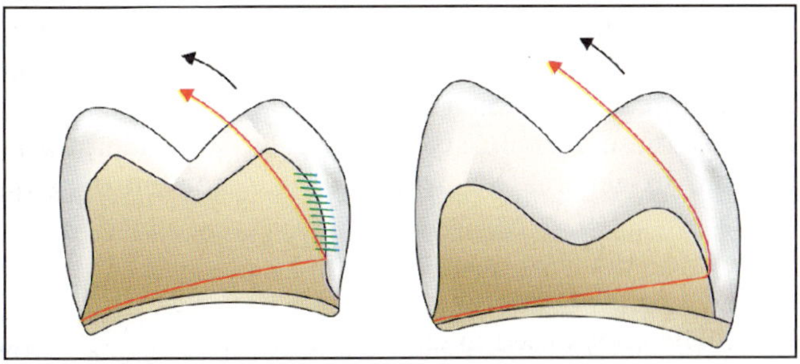

Fig. 10.9: Short preparations do not resist displacement compared to tall ones that have resistance areas (shaded in green)

- *Addition of pins and grooves:* Short preparations increase resistance by reducing the length of the arc of rotation (Fig. 10.10).

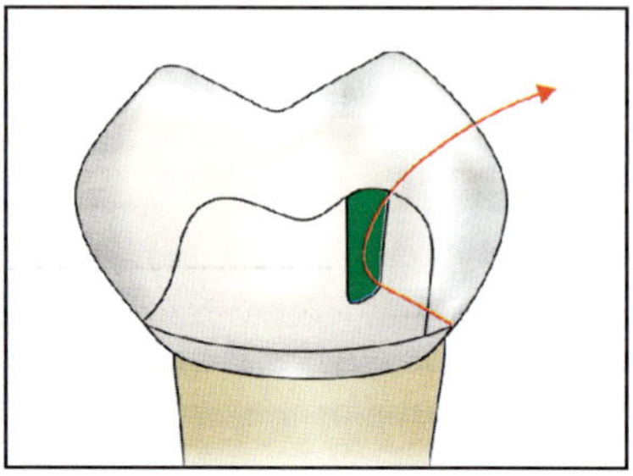

Fig. 10.10: Arc of rotation—in red

- In partial coverage restorations, *having grooves with walls perpendicular* to the direction of applied force increases the resistance form.

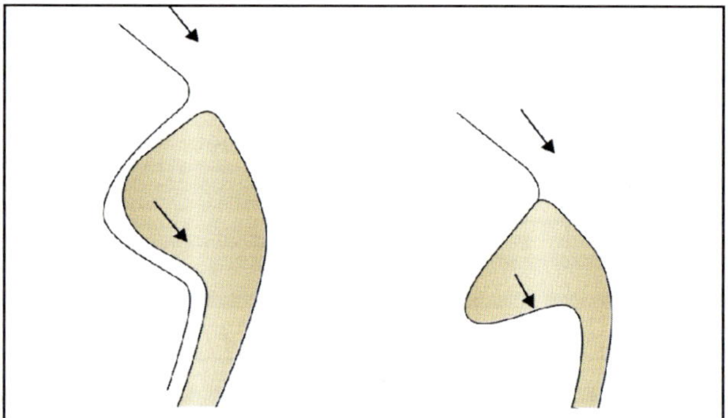

Oblique grooves do not offer resistance

Grooves with perpendicular walls offer resistance to movement

Fig. 10.11

- *Luting agent:* A luting agent with high compressive strength and modulus of elasticity are preferable. When subjected to other than long axis parallel forces, the cements are placed under compression. They should resist these compressive forces without undergoing plastic deformation. In general, the adhesive resin cement displays these properties.

3. Resistance to Deformation

- *Alloy type*: The alloys used in cast restorations should have sufficient strength. The base metal alloys are preferred over the gold alloys especially in long span FPD.

- *Alloy thickness:* Minimal thickness is essential for any alloy to have strength. It is suggested that the thickness should be at least 1.5 mm on centric cusps and 1mm on non-centric cusps. Uniform reduction with preservation of anatomy adds to the strength of the restoration because of the "corrugated effect"[15] of the planes (Fig. 10.12).

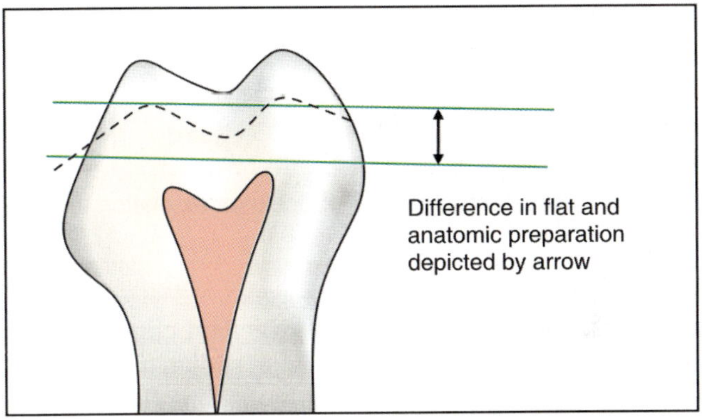

Fig. 10.12: Occlusal reduction for corrugated effect

- *Margin bulk:* Tooth reduction in the margin area should provide for adequate bulk of metal to prevent distortion.
- *Functional cusp bevel:* A wide bevel on the functional cusps provides space for an adequate bulk of metal in the area of heavy occlusal contact, thus reducing deformation of restoration (Fig. 10.13).

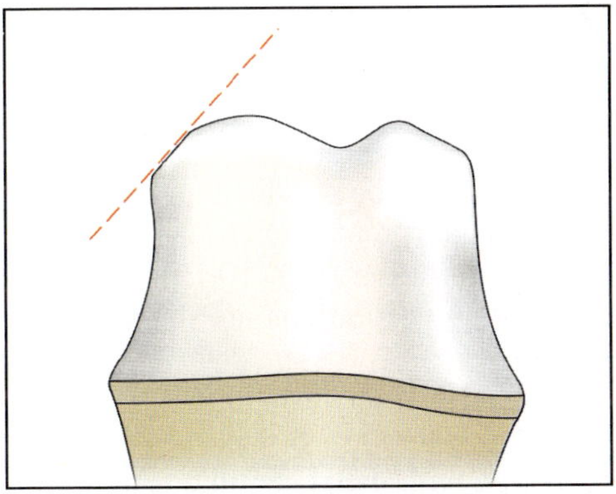

Fig. 10.13: Functional cusp bevel on mandibular molar

- *Margin location:* There should be no occlusal contact in the margin area. The margins of onlays and other partial coverage restorations should be placed beyond the area of centric contact (Fig. 10.14).

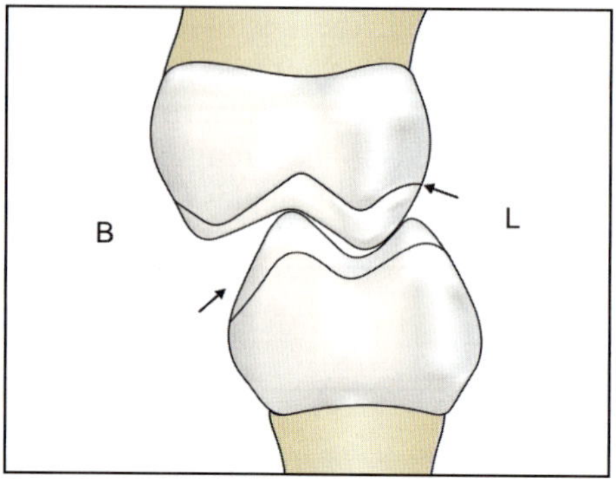

Fig. 10.14: Cross-sectional view of occlusal extension in onlays

ESTHETIC CONSIDERATIONS

Even when the treatment delivered is of excellent clinical quality, some patients will still be dissatisfied. The clinician should be able to recognize and satisfy the esthetic expectations of the patient. The various factors that contribute to an esthetically satisfactory restoration include:

- *Diagnosis:* Note down which parts of teeth are shown during smiling, talking and laughing. Some patients might not be satisfied with the metal not being visible only in normal functions and such expectations should be discussed and alternative plans arrived at.
- *Shade matching:* The color of the restoration should be matched accurately to those of adjacent teeth using shade guides. The provisional restorations can be of great help in this regard allowing the clinician to make small changes in the color periodically before arriving at the final shade of teeth. Sometimes, poor shade matching may be because of inadequate porcelain thickness and measures should be taken in this direction.
- *Shape of teeth:* Space should be provided in the preparation to properly shape the teeth. Inadequate preparation usually leads to improper shape and contour of the restoration (Fig. 10.15). The minimal suggested preparations for various restorations are discussed in the chapter on retainers.
- *Margin placement:* Supragingival margins may be practical only in cases of all ceramic restorations. Sometimes a collarless design may be used in conjunction with metal ceramic restoration. Metal margins must be hidden under the gingival crest with considerations given to periodontal health and biologic width. The margins should be designed to follow the contour of free gingiva for an esthetic result.
- *Partial coverage restorations:* the mesial margin should be placed just buccal to the contact hidden behind the distal line angle of adjacent

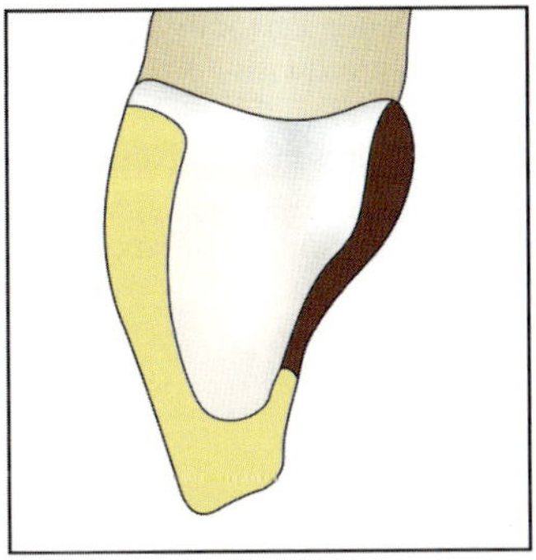

Fig. 10.15: Directions for minimal preparation in each type should be followed

tooth. The facial margins in maxillary teeth should extend just beyond the occlusofacial line angle with a short bevel to prevent enamel chipping.

When all the factors are considered together, the skilled clinician can prepare the teeth to accept a restoration that satisfies all the patient's needs.

REFERENCES

1. Rosensteil S.F., Land M.F., Fujimoto J., Contemporary fixed prosthodontics. 2001, 3rd ed.; Mosby, St Louis, Missouri.
2. Laforgia P.D., Milano V., Morea C., Desiate A., Temperature change in the pulp chamber during complete crown preparation, *J Prosthet. Dent* 1991; 65: 56–61.
3. Going RE. status report on cement bases, cavity liners, varnishes, primers and cleansers. *J Am. Dent. Assoc* 1972; 85: 654.
4. Perel M.L. Axial crown contours. *J Prosthet. Dent* 1971; 25: 642–9.
5. Sorensen J.A. A rationale for comparison of plaque-retaining properties of crown systems. *J Prosthet. Dent* 1989; 62: 264–9.
6. Bader J.D., Rozier R.G., McFall Jr. W.T., Ramsey D.L. Effect of crown margins on periodontal conditions in regularly attending patients. *J Prosthet. Dent* 1991; 65:75–9.
7. Felton D.A., Kanoy B.E., Bayne S.C., Wirthman G.P. Effect of in vivo crown margin discrepancies on periodontal health. *J Prosthet. Dent* 1991; 65: 357–64.
8. Shillingburg H.T., et al. fundamentals of fixed prosthodontics 1997. 3rd ed., Quintessence Publishing.
9. Wilson A.H., Chan D.C. The relationship between preparation convergence and retention of extra-coronal retainers. *J Prosthodont* 1994; 3: 74–8.
10. Reisbick M.H., Shillingburg H.T. Effect of preparation geometry on retention and resistance of cast gold restorations, *Calif. Dent. Assoc. J* 1975; 3: 51.
11. Smith B.G.N. The effect of surface roughness of prepared dentin on the retention of castings, *J Prosthet. Dent.*, 1970; 23: 187–98.
12. Saito C., Sakai Y., Node H., Fusayama T. Adhesion of polycarboxylate cements to dental casting alloys, *J Prosthet. Dent* 1976; 35: 543–8.

13. Ayad M.F., Rosenstiel S.F., Salama M. Influence of tooth surface roughness and type of cement on retention of complete cast crowns. *J Prosthet. Dent* 1997; 77: 116–21.
14. Parker M.H., Calverley M.J., Gardner M., Gundersen R.B. New guidelines for preparation taper. *J Prosthodont* 1993; 2: 61–6.
15. Guyer S.E. Multiple preparations for fixed prosthodontics. *J Prosthet. Dent* 1970; 23: 529–53.

11 Gingival Retraction

Achieving correct contours and adequate marginal adaptation of the restoration is essential to maintain tissue health after placement or cementation. Improper contours and defective margins lead to plaque retention resulting in localized inflammation. Proper contours and marginal adaptation is facilitated when prepared and non-prepared subgingival tooth contours are properly recorded in the impression. This is possible by displacing the gingival tissues away from the tooth surface temporarily, so that the impression material can flow between the tooth and gingiva for a detailed record. Such a procedure is called gingival retraction (Fig. 11.1).

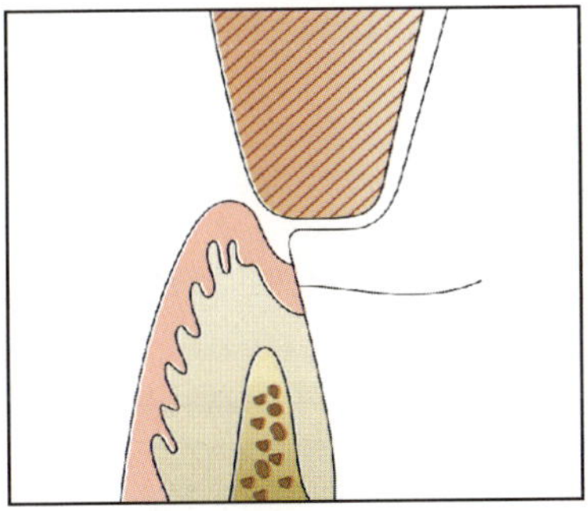

Fig. 11.1: Gingival retraction

According to Benson et al.[1] gingival retraction methods fall into:

1. Simple mechanical
2. Chemical-mechanical
3. Rotary gingival curettage
4. Election-surgical methods

The various methods can also be grouped into:

1. Mechanical
2. Chemico-mechanical
3. Chemical

4. Surgical:
   - Gingivectomy
   - Rotary curettage/gingitage
   - Electrosurgical
   - Laser surgery

MECHANICAL RETRACTION

I. Oversized Copper Bands

- Uses oversized copper bands contoured like the gingival margin and bent towards the margin of the preparation.
- A thread passing through the vents made in the copper band is used to pull the band after impression.
- A plug made of impression compound or self-cure resin restricts the impression material.
- The copper band must be gently but firmly placed over the tooth.

Darby and Darby[2] have described the advantages of copper band retraction as:

1. Tissue retraction is maximal
2. Deep subgingival margins may be recorded.
3. Reduced voids
4. Close adaptation to soft tissues
5. Sectional or full arch impressions may be made.
6. Only tray type material required.
7. Not required to pour the impression immediately.

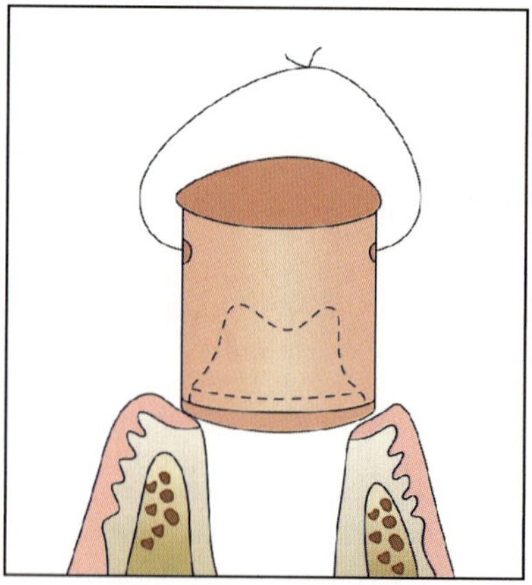

Fig. 11.2: Mechanical retraction

Advantages

1. Can be used in single unit impression.
2. Can be used to confirm margins in multiple preparations with one or two questionable margins.
3. Cost-effective.

Disadvantages

1. Excessive pressure during seating can lead to stripping of the tissues from the tooth.
2. Limited application.

II. Unimpregnated Cords

- Placement of unimpregnated cord is another method of mechanical dilation.
- Braided (Gingibraid, Vam R dental products), knitted (Ultrapak, Ultradent products), twisted or knitted forms of cords are available. The modifications are to make placement easier (Fig. 11.3).

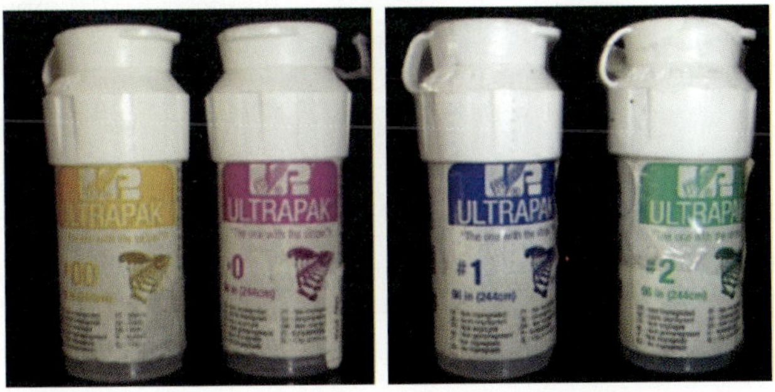

Fig. 11.3: Different sizes of ultrapak retraction cords

- Wool-like cords that can be flattened are available for placement in narrow sulci.

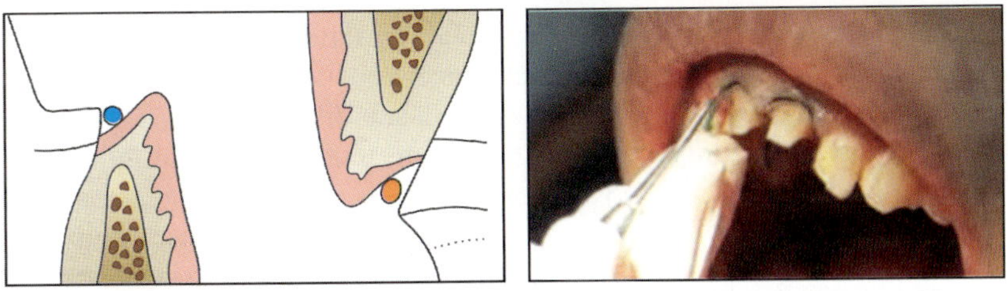

(a) Single cords placed in the sulcus

(b) Placement of cords in maxillary anterior region

Fig. 11.4: Unimpregnated cords

III. Application of Heavy, Extra-heavy and Special Weight Rubber Dam and Clamp[3]

- The rubber band compresses the gingival tissue exposing the gingival margins.
- When the margins are subgingival, the use of retraction cord between the rubber dam and the neck of the tooth may be necessary.
- The rubber dam is placed early in the preparation and helps a faster procedure as the moisture is completely eliminated from the area.
- It saves time.
- Less impression material is required.
- Disadvantages include
    a. It is impossible to record the shape of soft tissues in the impression
    b. Rubber dam needs to be applied for most teeth for satisfactory articulation of casts.
    c. When the rubber dam is in position, it is impossible to check the inter-arch distance (Fig. 11.5).

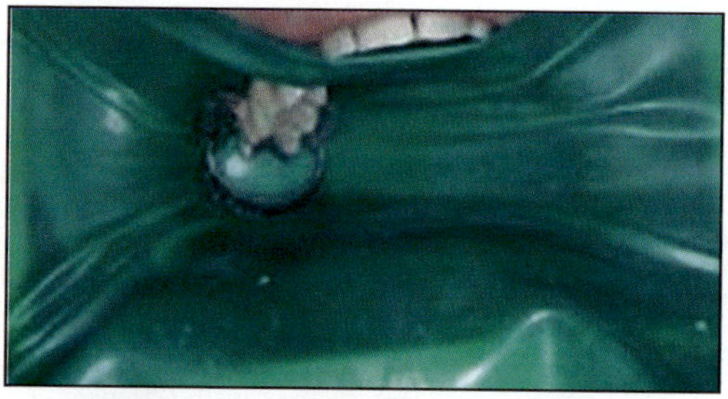

Fig. 11.5: Rubber dam in position

IV. Aluminum Shell

Use similar to copper band.

CHEMICO-MECHANICAL

- Most widely used method[4] of gingival retraction.
- Cords impregnated with chemicals or hemostatics is the most widely used chemico-mechanical method of tissue dilation.
- The most commonly used chemicals are aluminum chloride ($AlCl_3$) and ferric sulphate [$Fe_2(SO_4)_3$].
- The mechanism of action is that these astringents cause temporary reduced blood flow to the tissues causing shrinkage and reduced seepage of gingival fluid.
- The shrunken tissues expose the margins while reduced seepage allows better flow of the impression material.

- Cords pre-impregnated with epinephrine are available for use for retraction.
- Caution must be taken while using epinephrine as it is known to cause tachycardia specially when placed in lacerated tissue.[5]
- General anesthetics like halothane sensitize the myocardium to epinephrine and may produce life-threatening reactions. Hence, epinephrine should not be used under GA.
- Drugs available as non-prescription nasal decongestants and eye-washes have been evaluated.[6] Some of them have been found to be beneficial. However, further studies may be required before their use can be included in daily practice.

Requirements of Gingival Retraction Agent[4]

1. Should be effective in causing retraction
2. Should be safe locally and systemically
3. Effects should be spontaneously reversible
4. Should leave no permanent displacement

The Various Chemicals Available for use[6]

1. Racemic epinephrine –0.1% solution or 8% impregnated cord Mechanism of action—Vasoconstrictor
2. Aluminum chloride—5% or 25%
3. Ferric sulfate 13 to 20%—acts as a clotting agent. Often when the cord is removed, the clot is pulled out with it, and hemorrhage begins again. It does not cause actual shrinkage of tissues.
4. Alum—acts mainly as an astringent. It is safe and moderately effective.

Technique of Chemico-mechanical Retraction

- When the cord is used with impregnating solution, dip the cord, in the solution and squeeze out the excess solution.
- Impregnated cards may be moistened with water or normal tissue moisture to soften the cord, activate the chemical and also to prevent the cord from sticking to the thin epithelium and tearing it while removal.
- Loop the cord around the tooth and gently push it into the sulcus, using a suitable instrument (Fig. 11.1).
- The instrument should be angled towards the tooth and towards any cord already in position.
- Start in the inter-proximal area and encircle the tooth. Overlapping the cord at the end is advisable.

Double-cord technique: Two cords are placed into the same sulcus to achieve retraction. A thinner cord is placed into the sulcus first without overlap. This is followed by a thicker second one (Fig. 11.6). The second cord is usually removed before impression making.

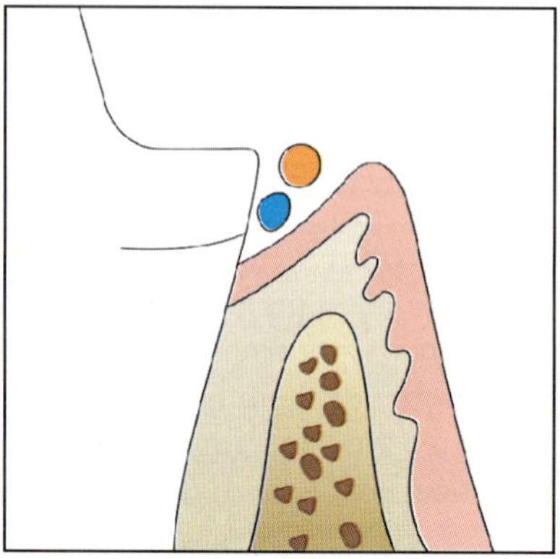

Fig. 11.6: Dual cord technique—schematic representation

Advantages

1. Adequate retraction with cleaner area (i.e. reduced bleeding and seepage)
2. Reliable method

Disadvantages

1. Cost of material.
2. Over packing can lead to tearing of gingival attachment.
3. Repeated use of displacement cord can cause gingival recession
4. Concern about chemical action on tooth surface—prolonged exposure of ferric sulfate has shown removal of smear layer and etching of peritubular dentin on the prepared tooth surface.[7]

CHEMICAL-RETRACTION

- Various chemicals like sulfuric and trichloroacetic acid, negatol[8] and zinc chloride[9] have been tried as gingival retraction agents in the past.
- Their undesirable effects on the gingiva led to their abandonment.
- The technique involves dipping of blade of the instrument in the chemical and placing it in the sulcus.
- It provides very minimal displacement.

SURGICAL

1. Conventional/Periodontal Surgery (Gingivectomy)

- It is used in cases of gingival hypertrophy, extensive tooth fracture that extends subgingivally.
- A more detailed discussion is available in the chapter on periodontal considerations.

- When this method is used, a provisional restoration is given until complete healing and then a more definitive restoration planned.

2. Electrosurgery

- Electrosurgery may be used in prosthodontics to[10,11]
  a. Remove redundant tissue to gain access for tooth preparation.
  b. Develop a trough around the prepared tooth for accurate impression.
  c. Control hemorrhage
  d. Remove opercula
  e. Plane and reshape tissue of an edentulous area for hygienic or ovate pontic.
- Requires healthy tissues; otherwise significant changes in gingival form or height may occur on healing.
- Contraindicated in patients with any electronic medical device (e.g. pacemaker) and in patients with delayed healing.
- Should not be used with metallic instruments.
- Should not contact metallic restorations as it can lead to irreversible pulp damage.
- A thin tip removes sulcular epithelium; tip may be angled 15° to 20° to remove a bulk of tissue based on requirement of the particular case.
- Tip should not contact the tooth or bone.
- Alternating current is generally used.
- A cutting stroke should not be repeated within 5 seconds. This is to permit heat dissipation.
- The sulcus is swabbed with hydrogen peroxide before a cord is placed.
- The recommended sequence of strokes for electrosurgery is lingual followed by buccal, mesial and distal (Fig. 11.7).

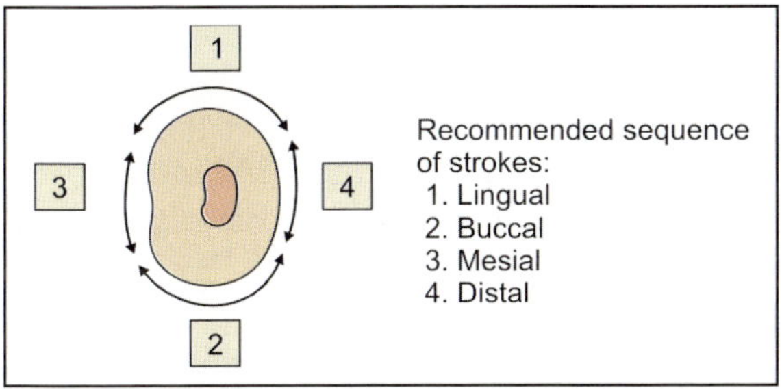

Fig. 11.7: Sequence of strokes

Advantages

1. Effective and easy removal.
2. Less postoperative pain.

3. Healing by primary intention—no scarring.
4. Atraumatic cutting of tissue.
5. Sterilizes the wound immediately.
6. No hemorrhage.

Disadvantages

1. Equipment cost.
2. Requires profound local anesthesia.
3. Cannot be used in all conditions.
4. Tissue odor—removal requires ventilated oral evacuation system.
5. Requires a skilled operator—cut only on the inner walls avoiding the gingival crest and epithelial attachment.
6. The electrode tip needs to be cleaned after each stroke—slow procedure.
7. Potential for gingival tissue recession.[12]

3. Rotary Gingival Curettage/Gingettage

- The concept was first described in 1945.[13]
- The technique involves the removal of epithelial tissue in the sulcus while a chamfer finish line is being prepared in the tooth structure.
- It is an uncontrolled procedure with reduced tactile sense.
- May lead to excessive deepening of the sulcus and bleeding.
- Should be done on healthy inflammation free gingiva.
- Induces recession of clinical magnitude (Fig. 11.8).[14]

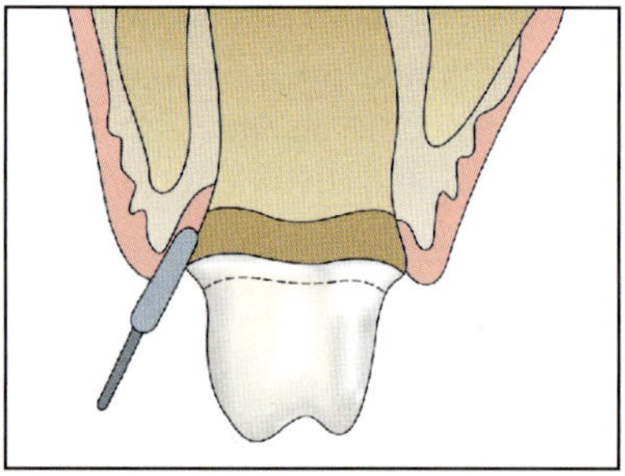

Fig. 11.8: Rotary instrument used to remove gingival tissue

4. Laser Surgery

- Recently lasers have been introduced for use in gingival retraction.
- Nd-YAG pulsed lasers are used.[15]

Advantages

a. Bloodless painless incision
b. Controlled tissue removal
c. Rapid healing

Disadvantages

a. Slow technique
b. Equipment requirement
c. Expensive

MATERIAL ADVANCES

Gingifoam

- It is a two paste system.
- The base paste contains polydimethyl siloxane and the catalyst paste contains tin.
- On mixing the two, hydrogen gas is produced resulting in foaming of the mixture.
- The foaming also enlarges the mix. This expansion is used to produce gingival separation from the tooth surface (Fig. 11.9).

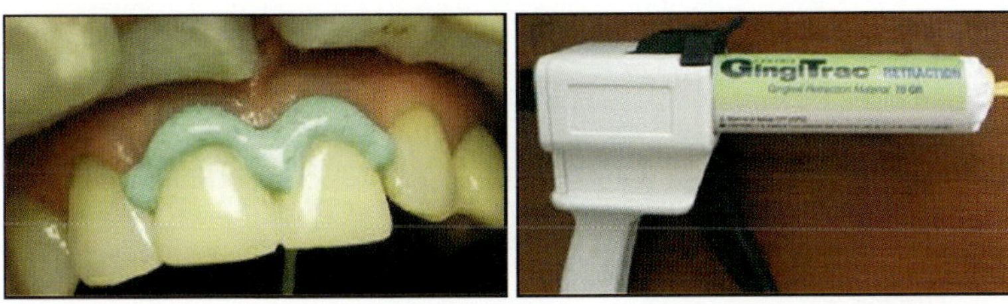

Placed into gingival sulcus Gun for placement of material

Fig. 11.9: Gingifoam

Expasyl

- It is a viscous paste of aluminum chloride, kaolin and waters (Fig. 11.10).
- It is delivered directly into the sulcus by a gun.

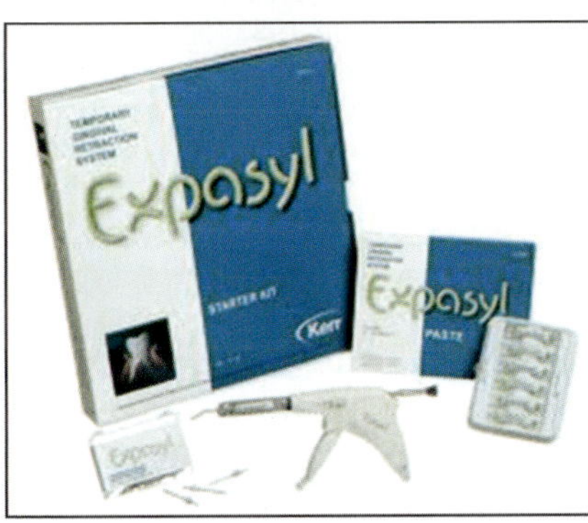

Fig. 11.10: Expasyl kit

- Minimal pressure is required for placement making it less probable of tearing the epithelial attachment.
- It is faster than cord placement.
- Controls bleeding and seepage.
- Available in different flavours.

REFERENCES

1. Benson B.W., Bomberg T.J., Hatch R.A., Hoffman W. Tissue displacement methods in fixed prosthodontics. *J Prosthet Dent* 1986; 55: 175–81.
2. Darby H., Darby L.H. Copper band gingival retraction to produce void free crown and bridge impressions. *J Prosthet Dent* 1973; 29: 513–16.
3. Elderton RJ. Rubber base impression over a rubber dam. *J Prosthet Dent* 1971; 25: 57–61.
4. Donovan T.E., Gandara B.K., Nemetz H. Review and survey of medicaments used with gingival retraction cords. *J Prosthet Dent* 1985; 53: 525–31.
5. Pelzner R.B., Kempler D., Stark M.M., Lum L.B., Nicholson R.J., Soelberg K.B. Human blood pressure and pulse rate response to racemic epinephrine retraction cord. *J Prosthet Dent* 1978; 39: 287–92.
6. Bowles W.H., Tardy S.J., Vahadi A. Evaluation of new gingival retraction agents. *J Dent Res* 1991; 70: 1447–9.
7. Land M.F., Rosenstiel S.F., Sandrik J.L. Disturbance of dentinal smear layer by acidic hemostatic agents. *J Prosthet Dent* 1994; 72: 4–7.
8. Benson B.W., Bomberg T.J., Hatch R.A., Hoffman W. Tissue displacement methods in fixed prosthodontics. *J Prosthet Dent* 1986; 55: 175–81.
9. Harrison J.D. Effect of retraction materials on the gingival sulcus epithelium. *J Prosthet Dent* 1961; 11: 514–21.
10. Patel M.G. Electrosurgical management of hyperplastic tissues. *J Prosthet Dent* 1986; 5: 145–7.
11. Podshadley A.G., Lundeen H.C. Electrosurgical procedures in crown and bridge restorations. *J Am Dent Assoc* 1968;77:1321–6.
12. DeVitre R., Galburt R.B., Maness W.J. Biometric comparison of bur and electrosurgical retraction methods. *J Prosthet Dent* 1985; 53:179–82.
13. Moskow B.S. The response of the gingival sulcus to instrumentation. *J Periodontol* 1964; 35: 112–26.
14. Azzi R., Tsao T.F., Carranza Jr., F.A., Kenney E.B. Comparative study of gingival retraction methods. *J Prosthet Dent* 1983; 50: 561–65.
15. Gherlone E.F., Maiorana C., Grassi R.F., Riccardo C. Franscesca. The use of 980-nm Diode and 1064-nm Nd:YAG laser for gingival retraction in fixed prostheses. *J Oral Laser Applications* 2004; 4:183–90.

12

Impressions in FPD

The various materials available for impression making in FPD include:

1. Reversible hydrocolloid
2. Irreversible hydrocolloid
3. Polysulphides
4. Condensation silicones
5. Addition silicones
6. Polyether impression material

A detailed discussion of each material is beyond the scope of this book and the reader is requested to refer books dealing with dental materials. However, a short discussion of advantages and disadvantages of each material when used in FPD is discussed followed by techniques.

REVERSIBLE HYDROCOLLOID

Advantages

1. Produce casts of excellent dimensional accuracy.
2. Good surface detail.
3. Custom tray is not required.
4. Can be used in mouths where obtaining a dry field is difficult.

Disadvantages

1. Requires immediate pouring because of poor dimensional stability.
2. May tear along the margins because the material is generally thin in the area.
3. Poor compatibility with die materials reduces surface hardness of the cast.
4. Lengthy procedure.

IRREVERSIBLE HYDROCOLLOID

Advantages

1. Fast—as it requires no pre-conditioning.
2. Easy to mix and load onto the tray.
3. Low cost.

Disadvantages

1. Does not record details adequately.
2. Can be used only for diagnostic casts (Fig. 12.1).

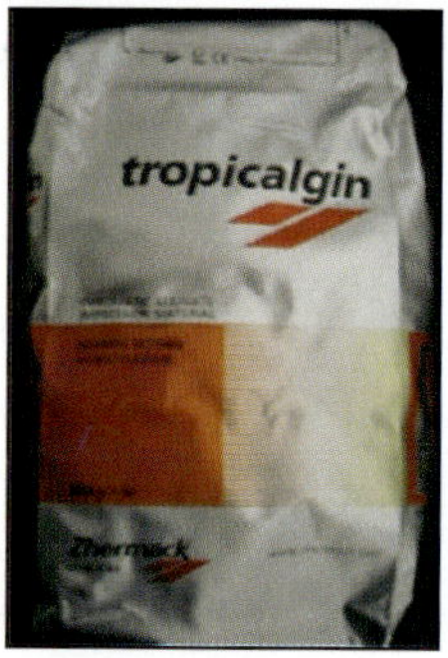

Fig. 12.1: Alginate impression material

POLYSULFIDE POLYMERS

Advantages

1. Does not tear, even in thin sections.
2. Better dimensional stability compared to hydrocolloids.

Disadvantages

1. Distortion/stretching may be unnoticeable because of high tear strength.
2. Should be poured within an hour. Keeping for a longer time may result in dimensional changes.
3. Long setting time.
4. Messy and has unpleasant odor.
5. Working time sensitive to temperature and humidity.

CONDENSATION SILICONE

Advantages

1. Dimensional stability better than that of hydrocolloids.
2. Short setting time in the mouth.
3. Less affected by high operating room temperatures and humidity.

Disadvantages

1. Poor wetting characteristics.
2. Low dimensional stability.
3. Difficulty to pour casts without trapping air.

ADDITION SILICONES

Advantages

1. Excellent dimensional stability.
2. Good elasticity—easy to retrieve impressions.
3. Delayed pouring is permitted and advisable, impressions may be sent to the lab for pouring.
4. Short setting time.

Disadvantages

1. Hydrophobic—but minimized by addition of surfactants.
2. Latex glove inhibition of setting—requires an assistant for mixing.
3. Tend to absorb moisture and expand.
4. Easy to trap bubbles while pouring.

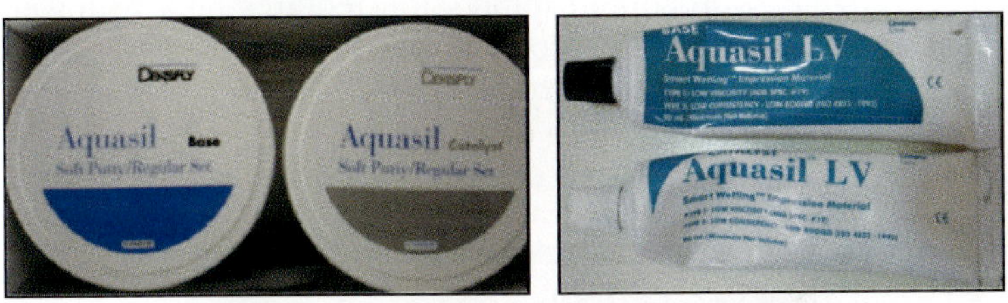

Putty | Light body

Fig. 12.2

POLYETHER

Advantages

1. Hydrophilic—does not require a dry field to record details.
2. Excellent dimensional stability.
3. Short setting time in mouth.
4. Easy to pour casts.

Disadvantages

1. Stiff—difficult to remove casts without damage.
2. Moisture absorption can result in significant dimensional change.
3. Short working time.
4. Some cases of allergy have been reported (Fig. 12.3).

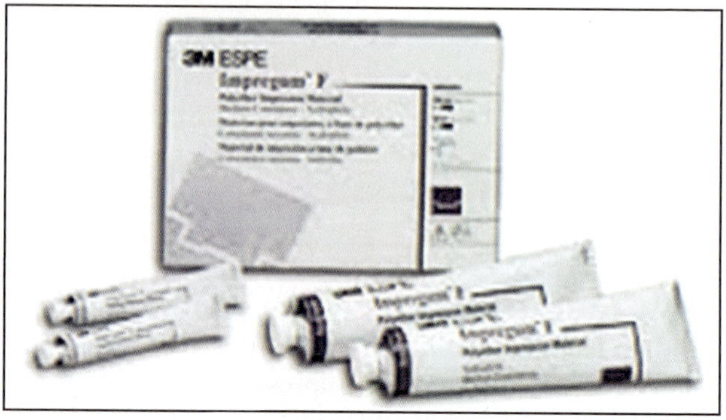

Fig. 12.3: Impregum impression material

TECHNIQUES OF IMPRESSION MAKING

Hydrocolloids

The irreversible hydrocolloid is used to make diagnostic casts only. The accuracy of the material / surface detail reproduction is insufficient for its use for working casts.

The reversible hydrocolloid impression requires bulk to lower the surface area/volume ratio to improve its dimensional stability. Therefore, its use does not require a custom try. Generally, a heavy body tray material is used with a less viscous syringe material. The syringe material does not require tempering (Fig. 12.4).

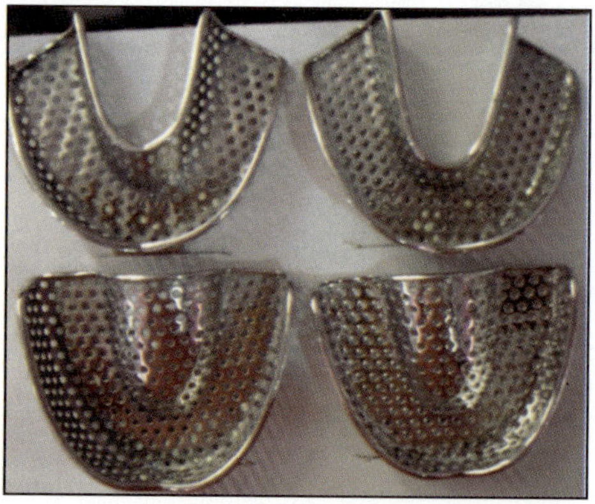

Fig. 12.4: Perforated impression trays used in making impressions

Once the retraction is done, the area is flooded with warm water. A dry field is not a must as the material is hydrophilic. The syringe material is placed around the tooth to be impressed first and then the whole tooth is covered. The tray material is loaded onto the selected stock tray. The tray is then placed into the mouth. The pressure of placement pushes the syringe material deeper and records the details in the area. The material is allowed to harden before attempting removal. Hardening of material is fastened by circulation of water for 5 to 6 minutes.

Non-aqueous Impression Materials

General Requirements

1. Custom tray—reduces the bulk of the materials. This reduces the stresses produced during removal, hence improves accuracy of impression. Reduced material also reduces polymerization shrinkage of the impression.
2. Follow manufacturers instructions for dispensing and manipulation. This reduces material defects.
3. Stops for custom tray—maintains the correct position while seating and correct thickness of material.

   The various impression techniques available are as follows:

1. Double-mix, single step technique

- A combination of heavy body and light body is used.
- The heavy body is mixed by the assistant and loaded onto the tray.
- The light body is mixed on the mixing pad and loaded into a syringe.

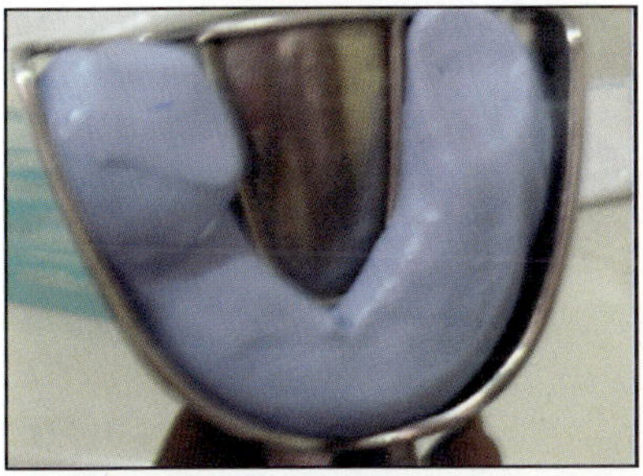

Fig. 12.5

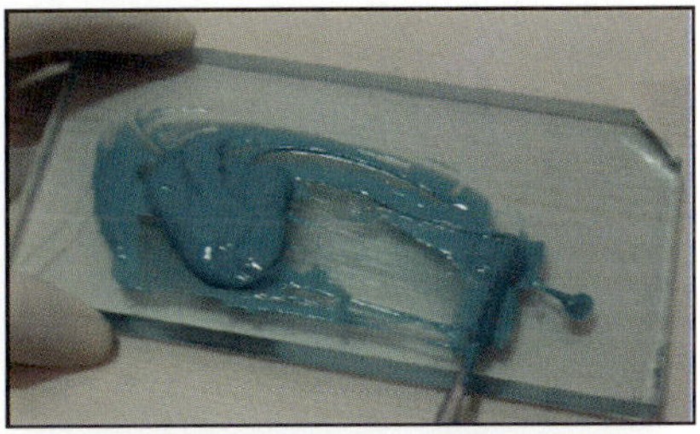

Fig. 12.6

- Remove the gingival retraction cord and gently dry the area with compressed air.
- Insert the tip of syringe nozzle into the most distant embrasure, touching the margin of the preparation.
- Slowly inject the material around the tooth so that the nozzle follows the material and never loses contact with the margins.
- Cover the axial surfaces of the preparation also.
- Thin the material by air blowing.

- Syringe material should also be placed along the edentulous areas, lingual concavities of anterior teeth (anterior guidance) and occlusal surfaces of posterior teeth (for accurate articulation).
- Seat the tray in the mouth and hold until the material hardens.
- Remove the impression and prepare for cast pouring.

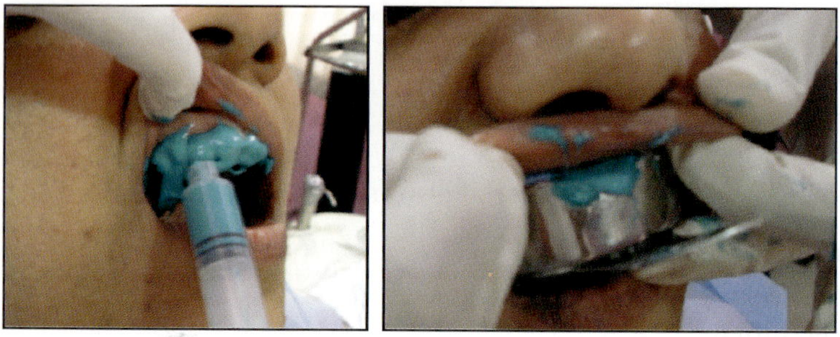

Fig. 12.7

2. Double-mix, two-step/putty-wash technique

- Most useful when an assistant is not available/trained.
- A combination of heavy body and light body is used.
- A heavy body matrix is obtained by making the impression before tooth preparation with or without the use of tin foil separator or spacer (Fig. 12.8).
- When used without spacer, space is created by trimming the impression.
- Once the tooth preparation is done and gingival retraction cords are in place, the light body material is mixed and loaded into the syringe.
- Syringe material is placed against the margins and prepared tooth as described previously, after removing the cord.

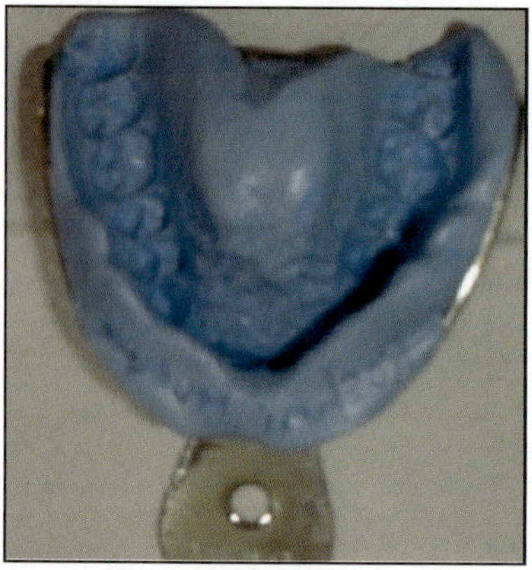

Fig. 12.8

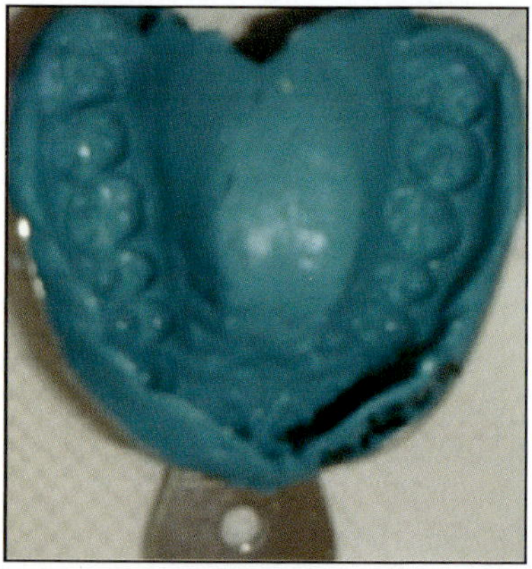

Fig. 12.9

- Part of the light body material is loaded onto the heavy body matrix.
- The heavy body matrix is now placed and the final impression is obtained (Fig. 12.9).
- The tray is removed after the material hardens and the impression is evaluated for accuracy.

3. Single-mix, single-step technique

- The technique is similar to double-mix single step technique
- The only difference is that only one mix is used to load the syringe as well as to fill the tray.
- Usually, the regular load impression materials are used in this technique.

4. Automix technique

- The technique is similar to single mix single step technique.
- The difference being that an auto-mixing gun-like device is used to mix the material.
- The tip of the gun is directly placed against the prepared tooth, as well as to load the material into the tray (Fig. 12.10).

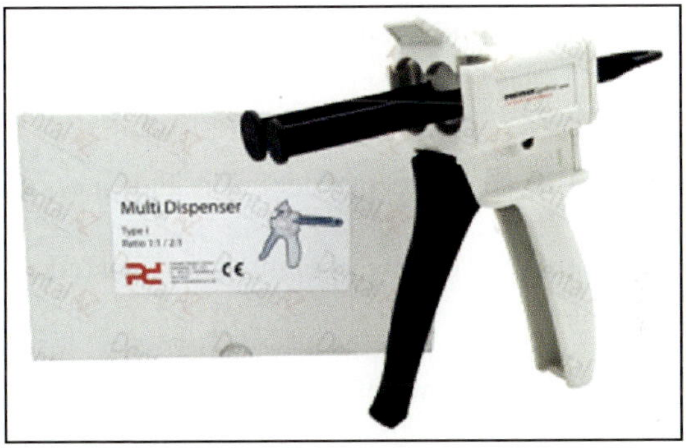

Fig. 12.10: Mixing gun for dual cartridge impression materials

5. Dual-arch impression technique

- Also called dual quad impression, closed bite dual arch impression, triple tray impression, accu-bite impression, or closed mouth impression.
- Usually a sectional impression of the side with the prepared tooth is made.
- The crossbar of the tray is fitted along the distal of the last tooth.
- The material is mixed and loaded onto both sides of the tray.
- In a syringe, load the material against the prepared tooth.
- The tray is seated upon the prepared tooth and patient is asked to bite on the impression material.

- Evaluate complete closure by checking inter-digitations on the opposite side of the arch.
- While removal, ask the patient to open the mouth. The impression adheres to one arch.
- Remove with equal pressure on both sides to minimize distortion of the tray.
- Prepare for cast pouring (Fig. 12.11).

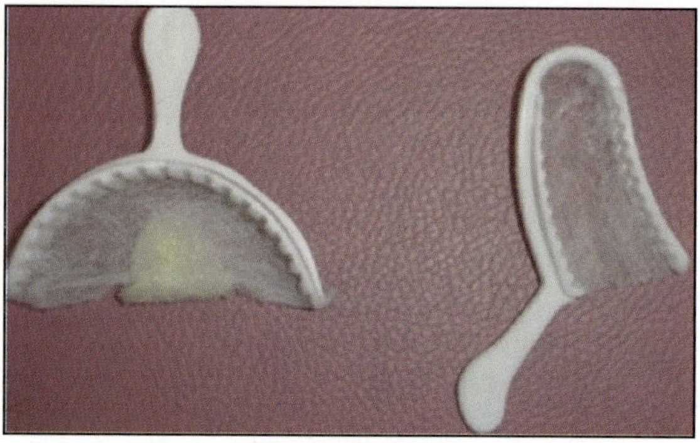

Fig. 12.11: Anterior and posterior dual arch impression trays

Advantages

1. Captures prepared tooth, opposing dentition and inter-occlusal record in one step.
2. Deformation of mandible during opening is minimized as it is a closed mouth impression.
3. Less impression material is required.
4. More comfortable for the patient.

Disadvantages

1. Success is dependent on rigidity of the impression material.
2. The shifting of teeth recorded in the impression is not accurate as it is a static impression method.
3. Technique sensitive, requires experienced hands.

BIBLIOGRAPHY

1. Anusavice K.J. Philip's Science of Dental Materials. 10th ed. W.B. Saunders company. Philadelphia, Pennsylvania.
2. Craig R.G., Powers J.M. Restorative Dental Materials. 11th ed. Mosby. St. Louis, Missouri.
3. Malone W.F.P., Koth D.L., Cavazos Jr. E., Kaiser, D.A., Morgano S.M. Tylman's theory and practice of fixed prosthodontics, 8th ed., All India Publishers and Distributors, Chennai, India.

4. Rosenstiel S.F. and M.F., Fujimoto J. Contemporary Fixed Prosthodontics. 3rd ed. Mosby. St. Louis, Missouri.
5. Shillingburg H.T., Hobo S., Whitsett L.D., Jacobi R., Brackett S.E., Fundamentals of fixed prosthodontics. 3rd ed. Quintessence Publishing Co. Inc. Carol stream, IL.

13 Luting Cements and Cementation

Once the prosthesis is ready, it needs to be attached to the teeth by means of a luting/ cementing medium. In fixed partial denture treatment, the cementation may include metal, metal ceramic, ceramic, composites, acrylics, laminates or pins and posts. The luting agents seal a space between two components, thus holding them together.

The cementation procedures can be broadly divided into:

1. Provisional cementation
2. Definitive cementation.

PROVISIONAL CEMENTATION

Provisional cementation is done so that the patient wears the prosthesis for assessment of appearance and function over a longer period of time by both patient and dentist. The provisional cements should adequately seal the restoration margins. The provisional cement should have minimal strength to facilitate easy removal. However, the strength should be adequate to prevent displacement during function.

The cements that are used for provisional cementation are:

1. Zinc oxide eugenol cements (with and without EBA)
2. Eugenol free zinc oxide cement.
3. Calcium hydroxide cements, e.g. Dycal, Reocap Temp
4. Admixed cements: Cements mixed with vaseline or petroleum jelly to reduce strength.
5. Composite cements (without bonding systems), e.g. Tempbond Clear, Provilink.

DEFINITIVE CEMENTATION

It is an important procedure and should be carefully done to ensure longevity of the restoration. Careful cement selection is essential to reduce margin discrepancies and obtain good occlusion. Removal of excess cement from the sulcus is important for long-term periodontal health. Attention should be paid to type of cement, manipulation and aftercare.

CHOICE OF DENTAL CEMENT

1. Type of restoration—conventional casting or adhesively bonded restoration.
2. Strength
3. Purpose—provisional or definitive cementation.

DENTAL CEMENTS

1. Zinc Phosphate Cement

It was first introduced in 1878. The powder contains zinc oxide (90%) and magnesium oxide (10%). The main ingredients of the liquid are phosphoric acid and water, with small amounts of aluminum phosphate and zinc phosphate. When the two are mixed, the phosphoric acid attacks the powder particles and releases zinc ions. Aluminum, which forms a complex with phosphoric acid, reacts with zinc and forms zinc aluminophosphate gel on the surface of remaining powder particles. Thus, the set cement consists of unreacted zinc oxide particles embedded in a cohesive matrix of zinc aluminophosphate (Fig. 13.1).

Properties

1. Compressive strength—96 to 110 MPa
2. Tensile strength—5.5 MPa
3. Mod of elasticity—13.7 GPa.
4. Solubility—low
5. Film thickness—25 μm
6. Retention: Bonding occurs by mechanical interlocking at interfaces and any coating applied on the tooth surface for pulp protection reduces retention.
7. It exhibits a low pH of 3.5 at the time of cementation. This property has been widely blamed for pulpal irritation by the cement. However, only the toxic effects of phosphoric acid are documented and not of zinc phosphate per se.

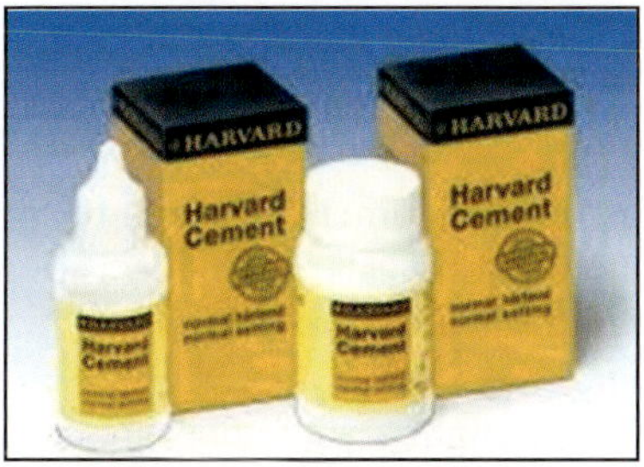

Fig. 13.1: Zinc phosphate cement

Zinc phosphate cement has a long history of successful use in prosthodontics. Even today it is the most commonly used cement for cast restorations especially in root-canal treated teeth.

2. Zinc Polycarboxylate Cement

The powder is similar to the zinc phosphate cement. The liquid is an aqueous solution of polyacrylic acid as a copolymer of acrylic acid with other carboxylic acids. This was the first cement system that developed an adhesive bond to tooth structure. Additives like stannous fluoride not only increases strength, but also contributes to fluoride release from the cement. When mixed, the acid releases zinc, magnesium and tin ions that react with carboxyl groups of adjacent polyacid chains to form a cross-linked salt. Microstructure of the set cement is similar to zinc phosphate cement (Fig. 13.2).

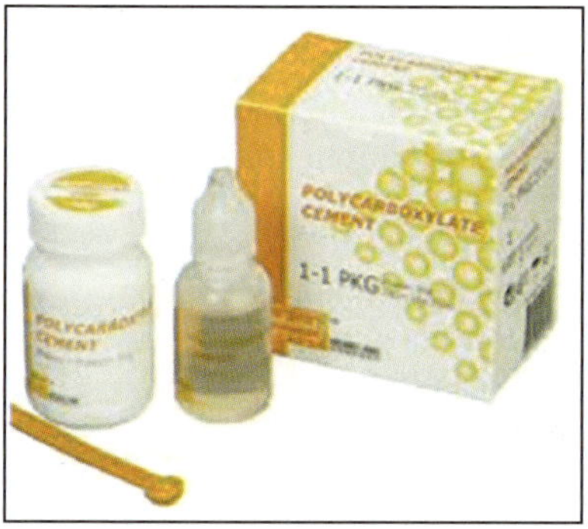

Fig. 13.2: Zinc polycarboxylate cement

Bonding to Tooth Structure

The polyacrylic acid is believed to react with calcium ions on the enamel or dentin surface via the carboxyl groups. The mechanism, however, is not entirely understood.

Properties

1. Compressive strength 55 to 67 MPa
2. Tensile strength—higher than that of zinc phosphate cement
3. Modulus of elasticity—2.4, to 4.4 GPa
4. Solubility—low in water, but increases when exposed to organic acid.
5. Film thickness—has pseudoplastic behavior. Though the mix is viscous, it undergoes thinning at an increased shear rate and yields a film thickness of 25 μm or less.
6. *Retention:* The bond strength to enamel is about 9 MPa and to dentin it is 3.3 MPa. The cement bonds to stainless steel but not to gold.

7. The pH of the mix is also low (4.8), but the larger size of polyacrylic acid molecule minimizes its penetration into the dentinal tubules.
8. Because of its plastic deformation potential, it is difficult to remove the excess cement after setting.

In clinical trials, the cement performs well or slightly better than zinc phosphate. However, there have been varying success rates, with claims of inferior long-term retention.

3. Glass Ionomer Cement

The powder is an acid soluble calcium fluoroaluminosilicate glass. The liquid is copolymer of polyacrylic acid with itaconic, maleic or tricarboxylic acids. Tartaric acid is added to the liquid to improve handling characteristics and increases working time. When mixed, the acid etches the surface of glass powder and releases calcium, aluminum, sodium and flourine ions. The polyacrylic acid chains are cross-linked by calcium ions initially which are later replaced by aluminum ions. The cross-linked phase becomes hydrated with the same water used for mixing over time (Fig. 13.3).

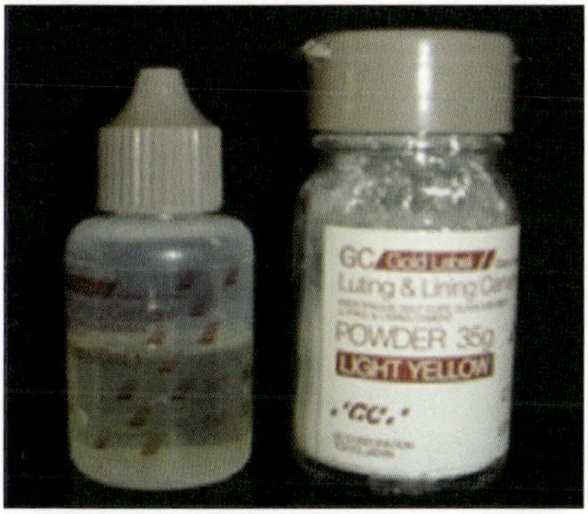

Fig. 13.3: Glass ionomer cement

Bonding to Tooth Structure

The mechanism primarily involves chelation of carboxyl groups of the polyacids with the calcium in the apatite of enamel and dentin. The bond is always stronger to enamel than dentin.

Properties

1. Compressive strength 150 MPa
2. Tensile strength 6.6 MPa
3. Modulus of elasticity 7.3 GPa
4. Solubility less than zinc phosphate cement

5. Film thickness – 24 μm
6. Retention: Bonds chemically to tooth. Bonding to the restoration can be produced by tin-plating the inner surfaces of the restoration. A tin – polyacrylic acid product overlying the tin layer on the restoration is formed.
7. pH is even lower than that of zinc phosphate cement during setting. However, the molecules of polyacrylic or polymaleic acid are large and are less likely to penetrate the dentinal tubules.

   The postoperative sensitivity reported with glass ionomer cement has been attributed to desiccation of the cement or bacterial contamination of dentin rather than irritation by cement. A calcium hydroxide coating is suggested for areas close to the pulp.
8. The set cement is translucent and can be used to cement restorations with porcelain labial margin.
9. Radiolucency makes distinguishing cement line from recurrent caries and overhangs difficult.

4. Resin—Modified Glass Ionomer or Hybrid Ionomer Cement

Introduced in an attempt to combine the fluoride release and adhesion properties of glass ionomer cement with higher strength and lower solubility of resins. They are less susceptible to early moisture exposure. However, they exhibit absorption and expansion and should not be used with all ceramic restorations.

5. Resin Luting Cements

The composition of resin cements is similar to resin-based composite cements. Resin matrix is formed by bis-GMA or diurethane methacrylate. The filler is inorganic with their volume less than that of regular composites and have a very low viscosity. These cements may be auto polymerizing for use under metallic restoration. They may be made light cure or dual-cure for use under translucent ceramic restorations (Fig. 13.4).

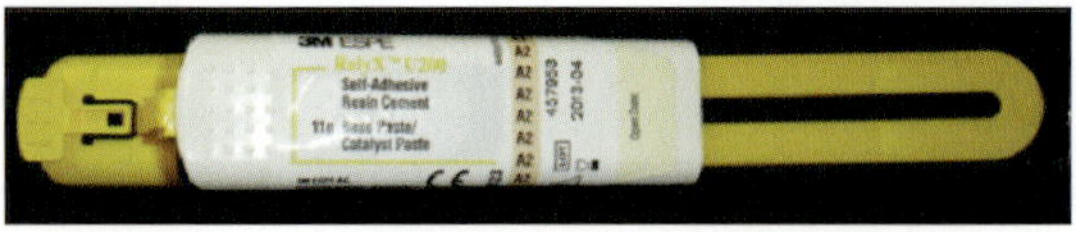

Fig. 13.4: Resin luting cements

Bonding to Tooth Structure

Micromechanical bonding to etched tooth surface and also to etched or pitted ceramic and metal restoration surface. The bond strength to enamel is higher than to dentin. Bonding to dentin might require the use of a dentin bonding agent.

Properties

1. Compressive strength—145 MPa
2. Tensile strength—high
3. Modulus of elasticity—2.1 to 3.1 GPa
4. Solubility—virtually insoluble in oral cavity.
5. Film thickness < 25 mm
6. Resin cements are less biocompatible compared to cements like GIC and severe pulpal reactions have been reported when applied to cut vital dentin. Dentin bonding agent may minimize such a reaction.
7. Their high polymerization shrinkage might contribute to marginal leakage.

6. Zinc Oxide Eugenol Cement

The main ingredients of this cement are zinc oxide and eugenol. When mixed, the zinc oxide undergoes hydrolysis and subsequently a reaction occurs between zinc hydroxide and eugenol to form a chelate.

The strength of these cements is low and it is used mainly as temporary luting cement. The marginal seal obtained is good (Fig. 13.5).

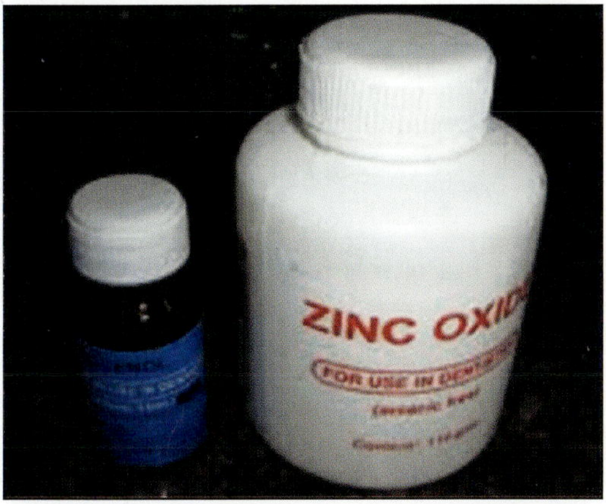

Fig. 13.5: Zinc oxide eugenol cement

Properties

1. Compressive strength 6 to 28 MPa
2. Film erectness 25
3. Solubility 0.04 wt%

The presence of residual free eugenol from this cement is thought to interfere with proper setting of resin bonded composites. Thus, there has been an effort to replace eugenol. The result is zinc oxide non-eugenol cement.

7. Ethoxybenzoic Acid Modified ZOE

A part of the eugenol is substituted with ortho-ethoxybenzoic acid and alumina is added to the powder. The properties of the cement are improved and can be used for a longer term (Fig. 13.6).

Properties

1. Compressive strength—55 Mpa
2. Tensile strength—4 MPa
3. Modulus of elasticity—5 GPa
4. Solubility—0.05 wt%
5. Extremely biocompatible.

The film thickness tends to be high and removal of excess is difficult. Hence, the cement use is confined to situations in which tooth sensitivity might be a problem. They may be used for short-term and intermediate term cementation of provisional acrylic crowns and FPDs.

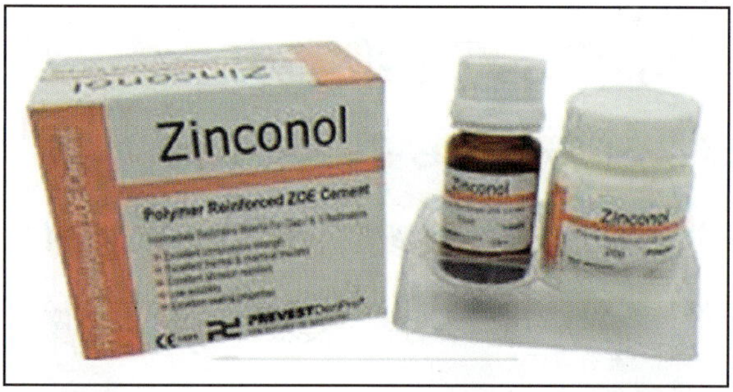

Fig. 13.6: Polymer reinforced ZOE cement

CEMENTATION PROCEDURE

The steps in cementation may vary slightly for different types of cements chosen.

1. Remove the provisional restoration and inspect all prepared surfaces for remains of provisional luting agent. Wash with pumice or hydrogen peroxide, if necessary.
2. The restoration surface is air-abraded, steam-cleaned or cleaned ultrasonically and washed with alcohol to remove any abrasive.
3. Isolate the area (with cotton rolls and saliva evacuator or rarely, rubber dam) (Fig. 13.7).
4. Any pulp protection required should be carried out.
5. Mix the cement according to manufacturer's instructions. Check the consistency by lifting some cement off the slab with the spatula. When the cement is of right consistency, it pulls into a thread of about 20 mm length before snapping back onto the slab.

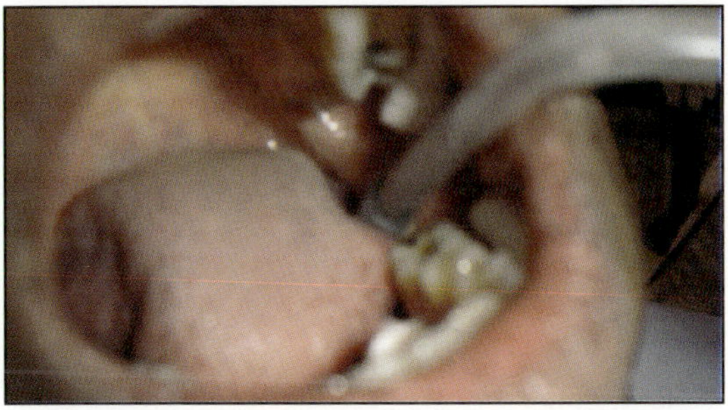

Fig. 13.7: Isolation with cotton rolls and saliva evacuator

6. Apply a thin coat of cement to the clean inner surface of the restoration.
7. Dry the tooth with a light blast of air and push the restoration into place by rocking it to apply dynamic seating force.
8. Check the margins to verify complete seating. Protect the setting cement from moisture.
9. Once the cement is fully set, remove excess cement. Early removal may lead to excessive removal with exposure of margins and increased solubility. Cements like zinc polycarboxylate and GIC tend to pull from under the restoration when not completely set. Hence ensure complete setting of these cements before attempting removal. Dental floss may be used to remove excess cement from inter-proximal areas.
10. Check occlusion with articulating paper or mylar strip or shim stock.
11. The patient should chew carefully on the restoration until the cement attains complete strength, i.e. 1 or 2 days.

Proper moisture control is a must for success of cementation. Any residual cement left in the gingival sulcus is detrimental to periodontal health. Ensure complete removal of the cement before the patient is dismissed.

BIBLIOGRAPHY

1. Anusavice K.J. Philip's Science of Dental Materials. 10th ed. W.B. Saunders company, Philadelphia, Pennsylvania.
2. Craig R.G., Powers J.M. Restorative Dental Materials. 11th ed. Mosby, St. Louis, Missouri.
3. Rosenstiel S.F., Land M.F., Fujimoto J. Contemporary Fixed Prosthodontics, 3rd ed. Mosby, St. Louis, Missouri.
4. Shillingburg H.T., Hobo S., Whitsett L.D., Jacobi R., Brackett S.E., Fundamentals of Fixed Prosthodontics. 3rd ed. Quintessence Publishing Co. Inc. Carol stream, IL.

PART IV
Miscellaneous

14. Provisional restorations
15. Postoperative care of FPD
16. Failures in FPD

14

Provisional Restorations

Fixed restorations involve lab procedures that follow the final impression before the final restoration is ready. In the meanwhile, a restoration is fabricated, for a short period of time pending a permanent restoration. Such a crown or fixed partial denture is called a provisional/temporary restoration. However, the dentist should not be lax about the quality of these restorations as they have to perform certain functions in the mouth. In case of a deliberate or unintentional delay in placing the definitive restoration, a provisional should be adequate to maintain patient health.

FUNCTIONS OF PROVISIONAL RESTORATIONS

A. Biologic Functions

a. Pulp Protection

In case of a vital tooth, a certain amount of pulp irritation is inevitable as the dentinal tubules are sectioned. Provisional restoration seals off this surface from the oral environment to prevent further irritation. If left uncovered, leakage through the tubules can lead to irreversible pulpal changes raising a need for root canal treatment.

b. Protection of the Periodontium

- A good provisional is essential for the health of the periodontium.
- Proper contours enable good gingival health. Overcontoured restoration can lead to gingival recession while undercontouring can lead to collapse of gingiva on the margins leading to tissue trauma during seating of the final restoration (Fig. 14.1).
- A smooth surface of provisional will limit plaque accumulation leading to better periodontal health.
- In an FPD the embrasures should be kept open. If it impinges on the gingiva, it may lead to inflammation and hyperplasia.
- Proximal contacts should be optimal as it is essential for the protection of interdental gingiva.

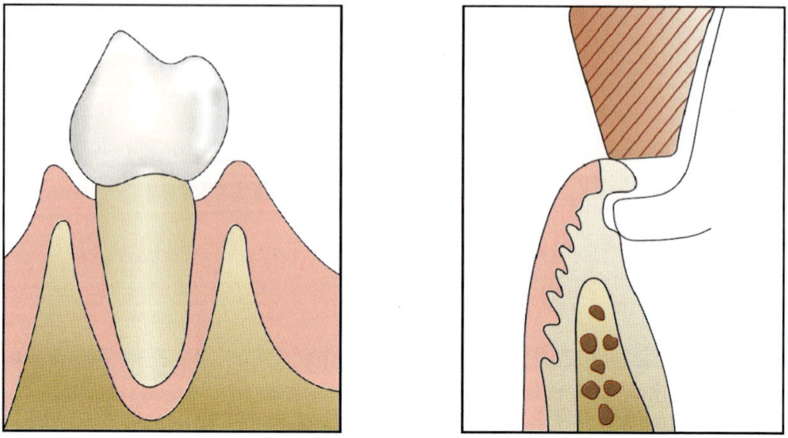

Overcontoured restoration leading to gingival recession

Gingiva collapsing onto the margins of preparation

Fig. 14.1: Protection of periodontium

c. Maintenance of Tooth Position

An adequate provisional with proximal contacts and good occlusion will maintain adjacent and opposing teeth in correct position.

d. Support for Muscles

A good provisional will support the cheek and facial muscles similar to the definitive restoration.

e. Protection of Margins

The provisional protects the margins of the preparation, so that the definitive restoration will have a good fit. Any chipping of enamel when left uncovered would compromise the fit.

B. Diagnostic Functions

- With the provisional in position, useful information may be collected regarding patients participation in maintenance of oral hygiene. The patient will maintain the definitive restoration only as well as he would maintain the provisional. The time may be used for patient education about maintenance.
- They give information about the correct tooth form and position for final restoration that would satisfy esthetics as well as phonetics.
- If the tooth has been out of occlusion, its reaction to placement of additional forces can be evaluated with the temporary.
- Reaction of bone to additional stresses on the abutment may also be evaluated with the provisional restorations.

- In case of a full mouth rehabilitation, temporaries help evaluate the acceptability of a new vertical dimension and occlusion to the muscles and the TMJ.

C. Mechanical Functions

1. Mastication

- During chewing, the provisional is expected to tolerate as much stresses as the definitive restoration. The provisional should function similar to its definitive counterpart aiding in chewing.

2. Removal without Fracture

- It should be possible to remove the provisional without fracture for reuse if needed. Procedures like metal try-in and Bisque trial require the provisional to be removed and then recemented.

D. Esthetic Functions

- Very important when placed in the visible area of the mouth.
- The color and translucency should be matched to the adjacent teeth.
- The provisional can often be used as a guide to achieve optimum esthetics in the permanent restoration, with proper tooth form, arrangement and lip support being finalized in the provisional and then adapted in the final restoration.

TECHNIQUES FOR FABRICATION

There are three techniques that are commonly used:

1. Indirect
2. Direct
3. Indirect–direct

Indirect Technique

- This technique is superior to direct technique.
- An impression is made of the prepared tooth/teeth and edentulous area.
- Cast is poured and undercuts blocked with plaster of Paris.
- Separating media is applied on the cast.
- When the matrix of external tooth surface is available, auto polymerizing resin is filled into the matrix.
- When the material reaches the dough stage, the matrix is gently but firmly placed on the cast.
- It is allowed to polymerize on the cast as tissue injury is not a concern.
- A rubber band may be applied over the matrix to ensure complete seating.

- The material may be bench cured or placed in a pressure pot with hot water at 20 psi for 5 minutes for curing (autopolymerizing resin).
- Davidoff[1] described an indirect method that uses heat-polymerizing acrylic resin. All steps are similar and the filled matrix is placed on the cast and placed in a pressure pot at 250°C at 30 psi for 30 minutes.
- The provisional is separated from the cast, trimmed, finished and polished.
- Occlusion is adjusted on the articulator.
- Provisional is placed in the mouth and checked for marginal fit, proximal contacts and occlusion.
- When matrix is not available, the material is placed on the cast directly and hand carved taking guidance from adjacent and opposing teeth.
- When adequate, it is cemented using temporary cement.

Points of Interest

1. Shillingburg[2] states that any vital tooth that is being relined should be done so via the indirect method because of the exothermic heat increase.
2. Moulding[3] found that the indirect method had significantly less marginal discrepancy than the direct technique that utilizes a pumping motion. Crispin et al[4] found that marginal fit could be improved by 70% using the indirect method to fabricate provisional restorations.
3. Chee et al[5] found that pressure curing polymethyl methacrylates reduced porosity and increased transverse strength when compared with the technique of bench curing.

Direct Technique

- Usually requires a matrix.
- Fabricated inside the mouth.

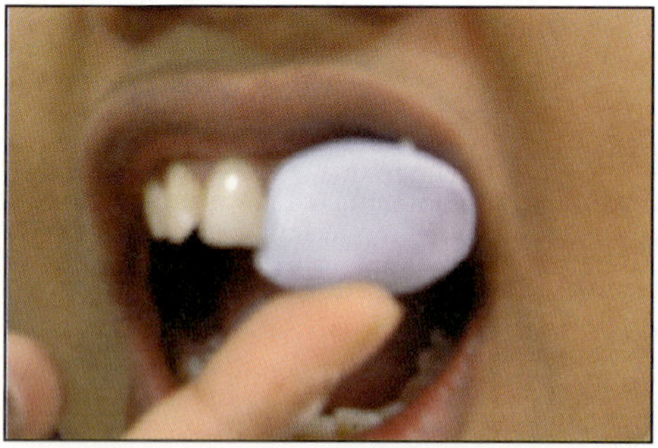

Fig. 14.2

- Loaded matrix is placed directly on the tooth; as the material reaches the rubbery stage, the material should be repeatedly removed and replaced on the tooth.

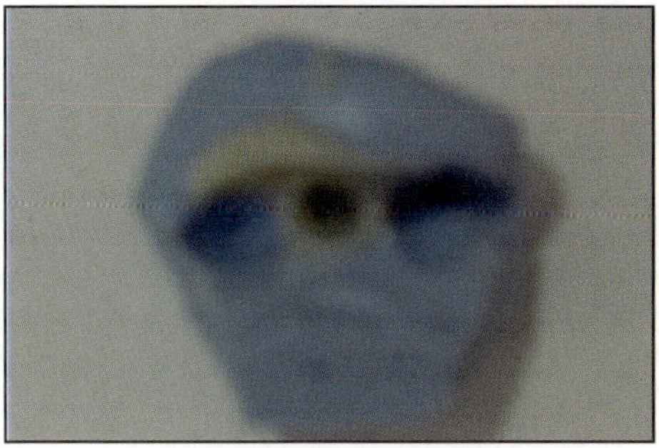

Fig. 14.3

- Doing this prevents the material from engaging the undercuts and also protects the pulp from heat of polymerization.
- Once the material hardens, it is separated from the tooth and matrix; trimmed and polished.
- Check for adequacy before cementation.
- Kaiser and Cavazos have described a technique in which wax is used to carve the missing tooth on the diagnostic cast and a duplicate of this is used to fabricate the matrix.[6]
- Nayyar and Edwards describe a direct technique for use with a single unit using a commercially available metal crown in which the crown is relined directly on the tooth with autopolymerizing resin.[7] Selection of the correct size and proper intraoral adjustments are critical.
- Christensen described another method for direct fabrication using wax impression of the tooth to be prepared and the two adjacent teeth as a matrix.[8] The technique is useful for single tooth restorations.

Indirect–Direct Technique

- As the name indicates, part of the procedure is indirect while part of it is direct.
- An impression of the mouth is made of the tooth itself when it is underprepared or of the mock preparation on the diagnostic cast.
- A temporary is fabricated for the under prepared tooth using the indirect technique.
- The tooth preparation is then completed in the mouth.
- The fabricated temporary is now used as the matrix. Its tissue surface is wetted with the monomer and lined again with resin similar to the direct technique.

- The bond formed between the two portions of the resin is a chemical bond.
- Cliché advocates spraying of water onto the abutment teeth to retard heat generation.[9]

The three techniques are compared with each other in the information box:

	Indirect technique	Direct technique	Indirect–direct technique
Advantages	• No contact of monomer to tissues, therefore exhibits reduced tissue injury. • Better marginal adaptation (stone restricts shrinkage of resin) • No distortion of resin as it is separated only after polymerization is complete • Patient is allowed to rest when the procedure is carried out by the lab • Reduced chair side time • Protection of pulp from the heat of polymerization	• No lab support or assistant training required • Faster.	• Less chair side time compared to direct • Lesser resin in direct contact with the tissues, hence reduced heat of polymerization • No contact of resin monomers in pontic area; hence reduced tissue sensitization/ allergic reaction • Part of the work is transferred to the assistant • Reduced occlusal adjustments as the patient can bite in centric occlusion while the resin sets • Improved marginal adaptation[10]
Disadvantages	• Lengthy procedure • Needs good lab support/ a trained assistant • Might require a time lag before the temporary can be cemented	• May cause gingival injury due to contact with monomer and pulp damage due to heat generation • Increased chair side time • Poor marginal fit • Resin distortion due to pumping action during polymerization[11] • Poor overall fit • Requires clinical skill	• Some monomer contact with the tissues is still present • Fabricated shell frequently needs adjustment

TYPES OF PROVISIONAL RESTORATIONS

1. Preformed, e.g. polycarbonate, cellulose acetate and metallic crowns
2. Custom made

Preformed Provisionals

Disadvantages

1. Usually need some form of modification like internal relief, re-contouring internal lining with autopolymerizing resin
2. Inferior occlusion with opposing dentition
3. Time consuming
4. Expensive
5. Usually used with single crowns only; not suitable for FPDs.

1. Polycarbonate

- Very color stable resin.
- Available in various tooth form, e.g. incisor, canine, premolar.
- Available in only one shade.
- Color can be slightly modified by the lining resin.
- Crown form becomes a part of the provisional.
- A tooth form is selected and modified internally, as necessary.
- The auto polymerizing resin is mixed and placed on the tissue surface of crown form already wetted with monomer.
- As the resin reaches dough stage, seat the crown on the prepared tooth directly or cast with gentle pressure to avoid turbulence.
- An escape hole may be placed on the incisal or occlusal aspect of the crown form (Fig. 14.4).
- Remove excess.

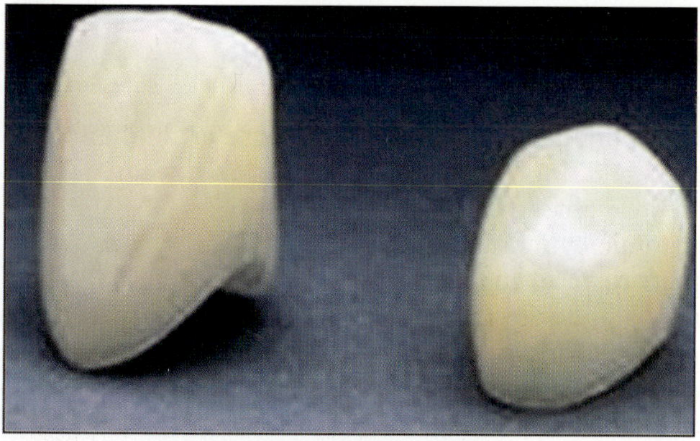

Fig. 14.4: Polycarbonate crown forms

- Remove and reseat the provisional several times as the resin reaches the dough stage. This ensures safe removal even in case of undercuts.
- Once the resin hardens, necessary trimming and polishing are performed.
- The provisional is ready for cementation.

2. Cellulose Acetate

- Cellulose acetate is a thin transparent material.
- Crown forms are available for all tooth types and varying sizes.
- The crown form is lined internally with auto-polymerizing resin, similar to polycarbonate crowns.
- Once the resin sets, the cellulose acetate crown form is torn off leaving the resin in proper shape, hence doesn't become a part of the restoration.
- Color of the provisional depends entirely on the color of resin.
- When the crown form is removed, the proximal contacts may be lost and some resin must be added in the area (Fig. 14.5).

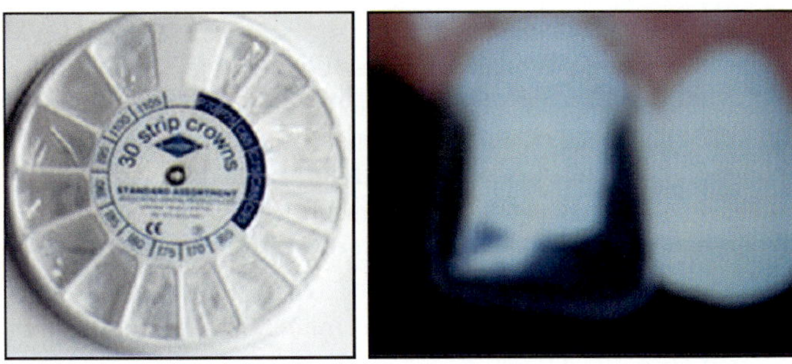

Transparent strip crowns

Fig. 14.5: Cellulose acetate

3. Metallic Crown Forms

Used in posteriors

- Nickel chromium shells are suitable for use in children only.
- Aluminum and tin-silver are used for posterior teeth.
- They are available in two forms:
  Non-anatomic/cylindrical forms
  Anatomic crown forms
  (a) Non-anatomic are inexpensive but require elaborate adjustments.
  (b) Anatomic forms are easier to modify to achieve acceptable occlusal and axial contours.
- Direct adjustment of the metallic crowns on prepared teeth should be avoided as the procedure can lead to fracture of prepared margin.

- These crowns form lack the rigidity for acceptable marginal strength and proximal contacts. They are rarely used in practice currently (Fig. 14.6).

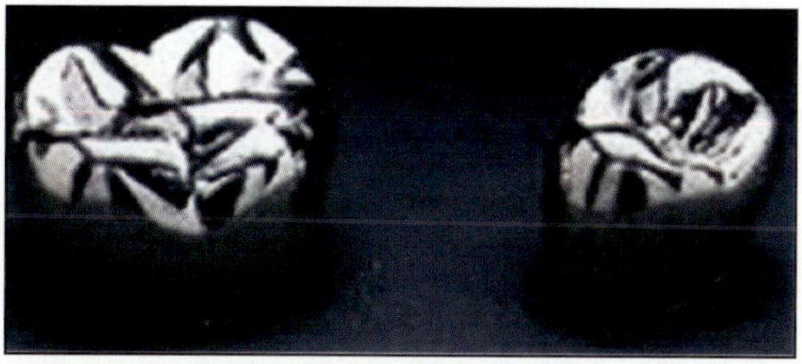

Fig. 14.6: Metal crown forms

CUSTOM-MADE PROVISIONALS

- The technique involves the use of a matrix prepared to replicate the external tooth surface.
- Into this matrix, a plastic material is loaded and placed over the prepared tooth to obtain the internal surface of the provisional.
- The custom matrix may be prepared from:
  a. Alginate or silicone putty impression made before tooth preparation or of a modified diagnostic cast
  b. Vacuum adapted thermoplastic sheet on a modified diagnostic cast.
- The most commonly used plastic material is autopolymerizing resin.
- Fabrication technique may be indirect, direct or indirect–direct (Fig. 14.7).

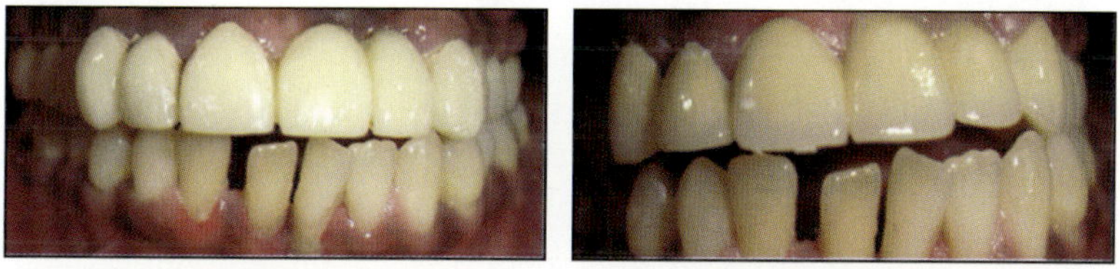

Custom-made provisional 6 unit bridge

Metal ceramic bridge with gingival porcelain in pontic area

Fig. 14.7: Custom-made provisionals

Advantages

1. Easy to fit—as it is made on the prepared tooth directly or indirectly.
2. Good occlusion.
3. Convenient and less time consuming.
4. Used both in single crowns as well as FPD.
5. Work may be transferred to the lab saving operatory time.

6. Expense of silicone putty is offset because it can be retained for a possible reuse later.

Disadvantages

1. Contact of monomer directly on the prepared tooth surface.
2. Heat of polymerization should be taken care of.
3. Monomer may injure delicate gingival tissues.[12]
4. Requires clinical skill.

MATERIALS FOR PROVISIONALS

The various materials available for use are:

1. Poly (methyl methacrylate) resin
   a. Autopolymerizing (Fig. 14.8).
   b. Heat polymerizing.
2. Microfilled composite.
3. Light-cured composite.
4. Fiber reinforced composite.
5. Cast metal restoration.
6. Epimine resin.

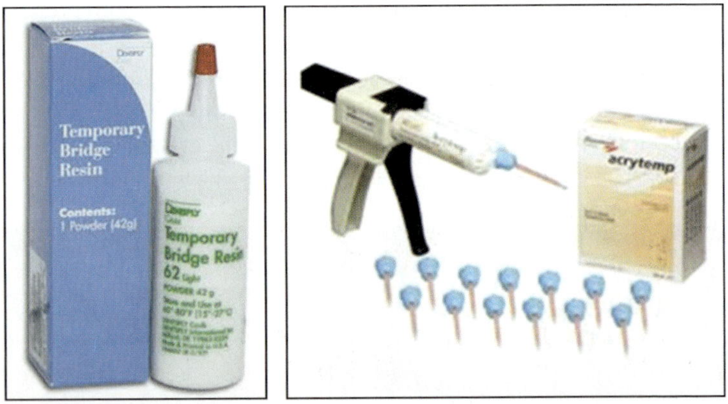

Autopolymerizing resin — Self-curing, self-mixing, composite resin

Fig. 14.8: Materials for provisionals

Indications for Fiber Reinforced (High Strength) Material

1. Long – span FPD
2. Purposeful delay in placement of permanent restoration.
3. Expected excessive forces on the prosthesis.
4. Breakage of other temporary material.
5. Highly developed masticatory muscles.

6. History of bruxism.
7. Reduced pontic space.
8. Small crown height.

REQUIREMENTS OF TEMPORARY MATERIAL

The requirements of a successful provisional may be accurately described as one that mimics the planned restoration(s) in occlusal and axial morphology as well as aesthetics, while fulfilling its requirements for maintaining tooth position and protecting the tooth structure during function.

1. *Strength:* Material should have adequate strength to resist fracture in use. Increasing bulk to improve strength is not a feasible option.
2. *Marginal adaptation:* Should be good. Studies have shown that materials display better marginal integrity while fabricated using indirect technique.[3,4,13]
3. *Color stability:* Temporary resins tend to discolor over a period of time. The epimine resin is very color unstable,[14] although it exhibits less exothermic heat during polymerization,[15] and better marginal adaptation.[16]
4. *Wear resistance:* Temporary restoration has to function as the definitive restoration. Poor wear resistance may lead to adjacent and opposing teeth movement.
5. *Odor:* Resins by nature are porous. They tend to collect deposits over a period and emit bad odor. It is preferable to have high density materials that are not porous.
6. *Easy to fabricate:* Should not require elaborate techniques for fabrication.
7. *Cementation:* Should be compatible with temporary cements. Methyl methacrylate resins are notorious for incompatibility with eugenol containing cements.
8. *Tissue response:* The material should not be irritating to the tissues.
9. *Ease of repair:* It should be possible to repair the temporary avoiding a time-consuming remake.
10. *Color matching:* Should be available in a variety of shades to obtain good esthetics.
11. *Polish:* The material should take high polish. This minimizes plaque accumulation.

DESIGN CONSIDERATIONS

The overall designing of provisional is very similar to the permanent counterpart, with a very few changes.

- Connector size must be increased in the provisional compared to the definitive restoration. This is to compensate for the strength of the restorative material. This is achieved by reducing the depth and sharpness of the embrasures. This not only increases the cross-sectional area of the connector but also reduces stress concentration due to sharp internal line angles.
- Pontic should allow for normal or enlarged embrasures and should not contact the ridge tissues with pressure. If so, hyperplasia of underlying tissues will alter the ridge form, leading to difficulty in seating the final restoration.
- Retainers are designed similar to the final restoration.

Various materials and techniques are available for use. The choice of material and technique should be based not only on scientific evidence, but also by what works best in the hands of the individual clinician. The ultimate goal is to fabricate a provisional restoration that is aesthetic, functional, and similar in contour to what is desired in the final prosthesis. If the clinician is able to achieve this in the provisional stage, achieving success in the final prosthesis will be much easier.

REFERENCES

1. Davidoff R. Heat-processed acrylic resin provisional restorations: an in-office procedure. *J Prosthet Dent* 1982; 48: 673–5.
2. Shillingburg H. Jr. Fundamentals of Fixed Prosthodontics. Third Edition. Berlin, Germany: Quintessence Publishing Co. Inc.; 1997.
3. Moulding M., Loney, R. Marginal accuracy of provisional restorations fabricated by different techniques. *Int J Prosthodon* 1994;7(5):468–72.
4. Crispin B.S., Watson J.F., Caputo A.A. The marginal accuracy of treatment restorations: a comparative analysis. *J Prosthet Dent* 1980; 44: 283–90.
5. Chee W., Donovan T.E., Daftary F., Siu T.M., The effect of vacuum-mixed autopolymerizing acrylic resins on porosity and transverse strength. *J Prosthet Dent.* 1988;60:517–19.
6. Kaiser, D., Cavazos, E., Temporization techniques in fixed prosthodontics. *Dent Clin North Am* 1985;29:403–12.
7. Nayyar A., Edwards W. Fabrication of a single posterior intermediate restoration. *Dent Tech* 1978;39:688–91.
8. Christensen G. Provisional restorations for fixed prosthodontics. *J Am Dent.* 1996;127:249–52.
9. Chiche G. Improving marginal adaptation of provisional restorations. Quintessence Int. 1990; 21: 325–9.
10. Barghi N. Simmons EW. The marginal integrity of temporary resin crowns. *J Prosthet Dent* 1976;36:274–7.
11. Fisher D., Shillingburg H. Jr. Dewhirst, R. Indirect temporary restorations. *J Am Dent* 1971; 82:160–3.
12. Waerhaug, J., Tissue reactions around artificial crowns. *J Periodontol* 1953; 24:172.

13. Monday J.J.L., Blais D. Marginal adaptation of provisional acrylic resin crowns. *J Prosthet Dent* 1985;54:194–7.
14. Crispin B.J., Caputo A. Color stability of temporary restorative materials. *J Prosthet Dent.* 1979; 42:27–33.
15. Braden M., Causton B., Clarke R.L. An ethylene imine derivative as a temporary crown and bridge material. *J Dent Res* 1971; 50:536–41.
16. Robinson F.B., Hovijitra S. Marginal fit of direct temporary crowns. *J Prosthet Dent.* 1982;47:390–2.

15 Postoperative Care of FPD

It is a general misconception that once the prosthesis is placed, the treatment is over. In fact, it is just the beginning of another phase of restorative care, i.e. maintenance/postoperative care. It is the duty of the dental team to see that the restoration functions as planned and remains useful for a long time. This as the aim, the postoperative appointments are structured to monitor the patient's dental health, motivate good oral hygiene habits, identify any new or recurrent disease, and render corrective treatment before any irreversible damage occurs.

GENERAL CARE

It includes overall care of the oral cavity. Any disease or predisposing factors should have been eliminated before the fixed prosthetic treatment is initiated. The mouth should be free of carious lesions and periodontal disease. The importance of maintaining a healthy oral environment should be highlighted to the patient.

1. Brushing

Good brushing habits are important. The brushing technique should be revised in every appointment. Deterioration of plaque-control efforts is common past the active phase of treatment and the dentist should be on a look out for such an event. The use of stains to identify plaque may be helpful in educating the patient.

2. Dental Floss and Interdental Brush

Both are important in removing plaque from inter-proximal areas where carious lesions usually begin.

3. Mouth Rinse

Use of mouth rinse may be prescribed to improve general oral health.

4. Diet

Any changes in diet, e.g. excessive sugar consumption, may predispose the patient to certain oral diseases. A watch on such changes and advise regarding same may be needed occasionally.

5. Saliva

It is an important consideration in oral health. Any drug leading to xerostomia should be monitored, as reduced saliva can lead to extensive carious lesions.[4]

SPECIFIC CARE

Abutments

i. Patient

- The health of abutments is of utmost importance for the well-being of FPD.
- Proper brushing around the cervical margins of the restoration must be demonstrated to the patient. The Bass or modified Bass technique allows proper cleansing as the bristles are directed towards the gingival sulcus.
- The use of inter-proximal brush is a must to clean the embrasure spaces.
- Any incidence of pain should be reported to the doctor.

ii. Operator

A keen observation for certain ailments is a must. These are:

I. Dental caries

- It is the most common cause of failure of a cast restoration.[1,2]
- At each appointment, the abutments should be thoroughly examined for any signs of caries.
- An explorer may be passed around the margins to assess early enamel lesions.
- Caries is most commonly seen in restorations with less than optional fit.
- Conservative treatment of caries at the cavosurface margin with amalgam, composite resin or gold oil may be possible for small lesions. Larger lesions may require replacement of the entire restoration.
- Root caries is another significant problem.[3]
- It is generally preferred to cover the exposed root surfaces with modified contours of the cast restoration.
- The focus should be on prevention, as the alternative usually requires elaborate procedure including a root canal treatment.

II. Pulp and periapical health

- When any pain is reported by the patient, the vitality of the abutment should be checked.

- Thermal or electric (contraindicated in full coverage restoration) may be used to determine vitality.
- Periodical radiographs are good indicators of changes in the area.
- It is a good practice to review teeth with fixed restorations periodically with radiographs. Any change is easily detectable by comparison with previous radiographs.

III. Periodontal health

- Periodontal disease is a common occurrence after placement of fixed prosthesis.[5]
- Subgingival margins, overcontouring and poorly fitting margins are associated with severe inflammation.[6,7]
- The patient should follow meticulous oral hygiene methods.
- The operator should keep a watch for gingival bleeding, furcation involvement and calculus formation as early signs of periodontal disease.

Pontics

I. Patient

When the sanitary and modified sanitary pontics are used, unwaxed floss can be looped through the embrasure spaces on each side, the loop can be pulled tightly against the convex pontic tissue surface and a sliding motion can be used to remove plaque. In case of modified ridge lap pontic, additional cleansing of the undersurface with an inter-proximal brush from the palatal aspect may be necessary (Fig. 15.1).

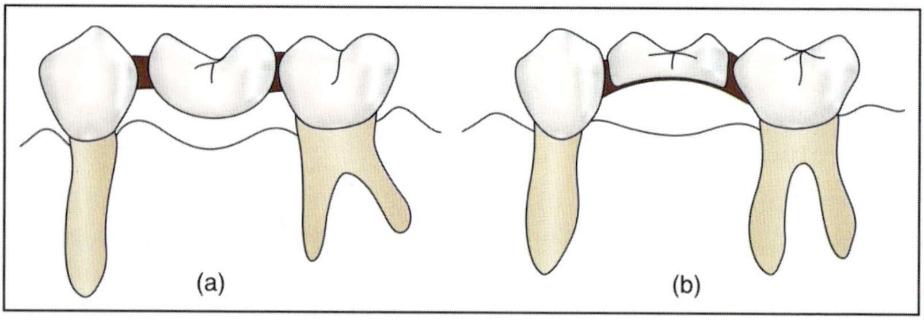

Fig. 15.1: Looping the dental floss to clean the undersurface is possible

II. Operator

Adequate designing of pontics eases the operator's job. However, an explorer may be used to detect deposits on the undersurface of the pontic and the patient educated on maintenance accordingly (Fig. 15.2).

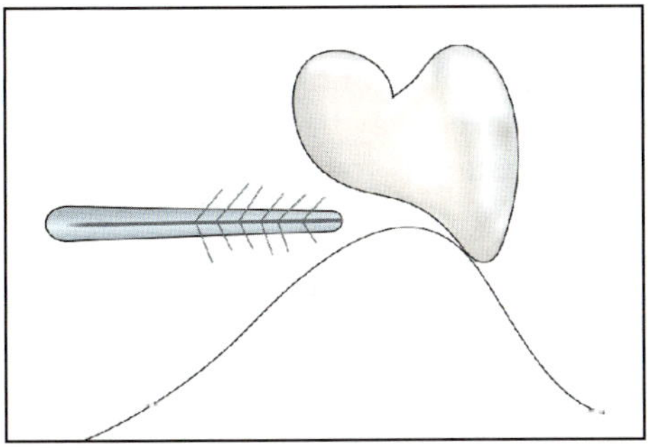

Fig. 15.2: Using an interdental brush to clean the gingival surface of pontic

Connectors

I. Patient

The loop of floss used to clean the undersurface of pontic can be extended to clean the undersurface of the connector as well. Use of inter-proximal brush in the area is advisable. Any pain during function may indicate fracture of connector and should be promptly reported.

II. Operator

- An explorer can be used to detect soft or hard deposits on the under-surface. Patient may require education about consequences of poor maintenance.
- When pain is reported and the cause is not obvious, an evaluation of connector fracture is required.
- When one connector fractures, the pontic is cantilevered from the other abutment, generating excessive pressure on the abutment leading to pain.
- Connector failure may be very difficult to detect clinically. A wedge placed to separate the individual components of FPD may help in correct diagnosis.

Retainers

I. Patient

- Specific care of retainer overlaps with the care of abutments.
- Cleansing around the margins of the restoration is of utmost importance.
- Any exposure of tooth following attrition of restoration or fracture of veneers should be immediately reported.
- Resin facings tend to absorb color over a period of time and the patient should follow the advice regarding colorant foods.

II. Operator

- Fracture of veneers or attrition of restoration may be treated with repair or replacement as the need may be.
- Regular check-up of margins for loss of cement or incipient caries is necessary.
- Every postoperative appointment should include meticulous scaling of the area.

REFERENCES

1. Walton J.N., Gardner F.M., Agar J.R. A survey of crown and fixed partial denture failures: Length of service and reasons for replacement. *J Prosthet Dent* 1986; 56:416–421.
2. Libby G., Arcuri M.R., LaVelle W.E., Hebl L., Longevity of fixed partial dentures. *J Prosthet Dent* 1997;78:127–31.
3. Gordon S.R. Older adults: Demographics and need for quality care. *J Prosthet Dent* 1989;61:737–41.
4. Gibson G. Identifying and treating xerostomia in restorative patients. *J Esthet Dent* 1998;10:253.
5. Valderhaug J. Gingival reaction to fixed prosthesis. *J Dent Res* 1971;50: 74–7.
6. Wagman S.S. The role of coronal contour in gingival health. *J Prosthet Dent* 1977;37:280–7.
7. Mojon P., et al. Relationship between prosthodontic status, caries and periodontal disease in a geriatric population. *Int J Prosthodont* 1995;8:564–71.

16

Failures in FPD

Non-performance of something as desired is termed failure. The process progresses through stages before it reaches absolute failure. At some stages may be repairable and is considered a complication.

CLASSIFICATION OF FAILURES

1. Based on the Severity

a. Mild—those that are correctable without having to remake the restoration.
b. Severe—those that require replacement of restoration with or without treatment of the supporting tissues.

2. Based on the Cause

a. Biologic
b. Mechanical
c. Esthetic.

3. J.J. Manappallil Classification

Discussed at the end of the chapter.

4. Based on the Procedure Responsible for Failure

a. Clinical failure—due to improper clinical procedures.
b. Technical failure—due to improper laboratory procedures.
c. Failure due to patient factor—systemic health of the patient and maintenance of the prosthesis.

BIOLOGIC FAILURES

Any change in the abutment tooth and its surrounding environment that might eventually lead to failure of a fixed prosthesis is called a biologic failure.

1. Caries

Dental caries is the most common cause of failure of FPDs.[1,2]

Cause

- Continued progression of existing caries due to incomplete removal.
- Secondary caries occurring at the margins of loose retainers.
- Cement dissolution at the margins of ill-fitting retainer (Fig. 16.1).
- Change in the patient's diet, or a lapse in oral hygiene.

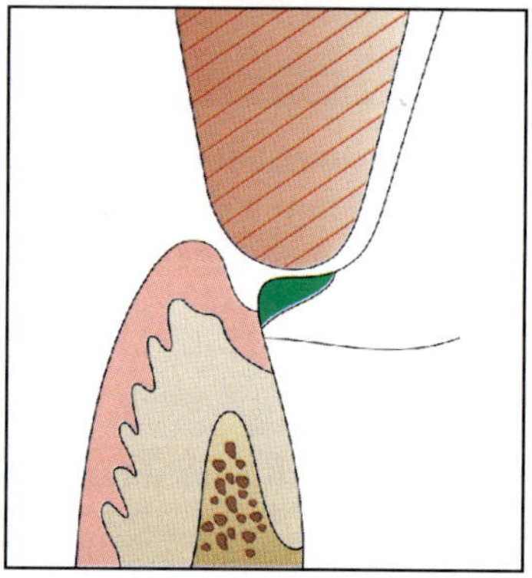

Fig. 16.1: Initiation of caries along the margins

Detection

- Early detection is possible mainly through comprehensive probing of the margins and tooth surface with an explorer.
- Radiographs may be useful in detection of inter-proximal caries.

Treatment

- Small carious lesions may be restored without a need to fabricate a new prosthesis. Gold foil, amalgam or tooth colored (in esthetic areas) restorative material may be used.
- Carious lesions in proximal surface may require removal of the prosthesis to obtain access.
- In small marginal lesions, the tooth preparation can be extended to eliminate the caries and a new prosthesis can be fabricated.
- When the lesion is large, the caries is excavated and an amalgam restoration done. The abutment preparation can now be extended to cover the filling, and a new restoration fabricated.
- Extensive lesions may encroach on the pulp making endodontic treatment necessary.
- If unrestorable, extraction may become the only choice.

Care

- Meticulous oral hygiene especially for patients with a high caries index.
- Fluoride dentifrices, mouth rinses containing fluoride and professionally applied topical fluoride.

2. Problems with the Pulp

Cause

- Excessive heat generated during tooth preparation that is not adequately dissipated.
- Caries beneath the restoration.
- Chemical injury from cements, retraction agents, etc.
- Preparation close to the pulp.

Detection

- Clinically, post insertion pulpal sensitivity on abutment teeth that does not subside with time or intense pain.
- Radiographs that show periapical abnormalities.

Treatment

- Endodontic treatment of the abutment is essential.
- RCT may be performed after removing the restoration or through a hole in the prosthesis. This hole can be restored with gold foil, amalgam or a cast metal inlay without the need for a new prosthesis.
- In cases of radicular retainer, the prognosis of the prosthesis may be reduced if the pin retention of a core is damaged.
- If the restoration is damaged or if it no longer satisfies the qualities required, a new prosthesis may become mandatory.

3. Periodontal Diseases

Cause

- Patient poorly motivated in maintenance.
- Poor design of the prosthesis.
- Altered systemic health of the patient.

Detection

- Clinically, check the health of the gingiva, probing depths, bleeding on probing and other indicators of periodontal diseases.
- Radiographs that detect bone loss, furcation involvement, etc.

Treatment

- Poor maintenance may be set right by adequate motivation and participation by the patient.

- Improved design of the prosthesis with emphasis on margin design and adaptation, contours, connector and pontic design and highly polished surfaces.
- Mild bone loss may be treated with surgery without the loss of abutment.
- If large amount of bone is lost, and the prognosis of the tooth is poor, the tooth may have to be removed and a new treatment planned (Fig. 16.2).

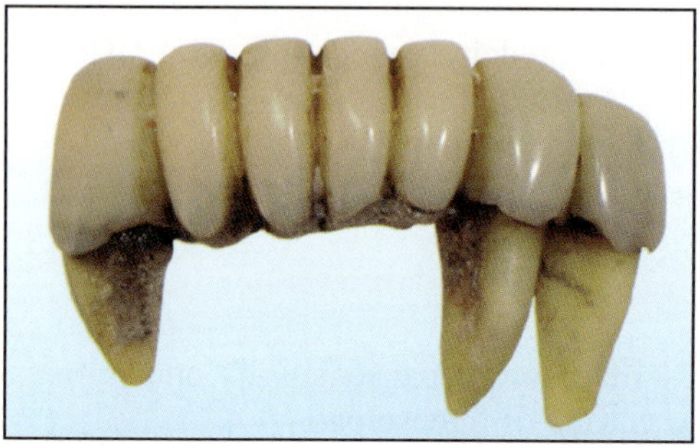

Fig. 16.2: Severe failure due to improper diagnosis, poor patient motivation and periodontal involvement

4. Occlusal Problems

Cause

- Interfering centric or eccentric occlusal contacts are the main cause.
- It can lead to symptoms like abutment mobility, periodontal disease, pulp degeneration, trauma from occlusion, perforations, neuromuscular discomfort and severe pain.

Detection

- Early detection is very important to maintain good prognosis of the prosthesis.
- Diagnosis is mainly by eliciting a detailed history and meticulous examination.

Treatment

- The interference can be eliminated by occlusal adjustment without permanent damage.
- In cases of excessive mobility or severe periodontal disease, changing to an RPD with bilateral bracing would be a better choice of treatment.

5. Endodontic Complications

Cause

- Incomplete preparation of the canal before restoration.

- Perforation of the tooth/root during preparation of pinholes for pin retained restorations.
- Perforation during insertion of pins.
- Perforation during post space preparation.

Detection

Detection is by clinical probing, radiographs and patient complaint of pain.

Treatment

- When the perforation is occlusal to the periodontal ligament, the tooth preparation may be extended to cover the defect.
- If the perforation extends into the periodontal ligament, periodontal surgery may performed to place a restoration in the perforation.
- If the pin projects into the ligament, it may be smoothed off and the restorations carried out as planned.
- Perforations in the furcation areas may necessitate hemisection or radectomy.
- In a vital tooth if the pinholes or pins perforate into the pulp chamber, endodontic treatment is mandatory.
- When the complication reduces the prognosis of the tooth, extraction and change of abutment may be necessary.

6. Movement of the Tooth

- The tooth serving as a bridge abutment may become loose, drift or both due to occlusal trauma, periodontal disease or relapsing orthodontic treatment.
- The cause of the movement should be ascertained and corrected.
- Some cases might require that the prosthesis is remade.

MECHANICAL FAILURES

1. Loss of Retention

Loss of retention is the most commonly reported mechanical failure.[1,2]

Cause

Poor retention form, excessive span length, heavy occlusal forces, flexible prosthesis, improper cementation, cement dissolution, etc.

Detection

- Patient reports of awareness of looseness or sensitivity to temperature or sweets.

- Recurring bad taste or odor that needs to be differentiated from poor oral hygiene or periodontal problems.
- Operator attempt to unseat the prosthesis by lifting it up and down will reveal that the fluid is drawn under the casting when lifted and forced out with bubbling when seated back.

Treatment

- Remove the prosthesis and evaluate the abutment.
- If both the restoration and the abutment are intact, the restoration can be recemented. Improper cementation procedure probably caused loss of retention.
- If the loss of retention is due to inadequate design, it has to be modified and a new prosthesis is made.
- In cases of repeated loss of retention, all factors need to be evaluated and a change in treatment plan considered.

2. Connector Failure

Cause

- Connector failures may occur between retainers and pontics or between two pontics. Failures may occur in soldered as well as cast connectors.
- Reasons may be an existing internal porosity, insufficient size, improper design, improper choice of solder, failure of the solder to bond to the metal, etc.

Detection

- Early detection is important because it leaves the pontic cantilevered to the abutment.
- Patient report of pain, clinically trying to separate the components of the FPD may aid in detection.

Treatment

- The prosthesis should be removed and remade as soon as possible.
- When a delay is anticipated, cut through the unbroken connector and construct an RPD.
- A repair may be attempted by preparing a dovetailed inlay like cavity in the fracture site, making an impression and cementing a casting into this cavity.

3. Occlusal Wear and Perforation

Cause

- Like the posterior teeth, the occlusal surface of the restoration wears down with normal chewing.

- Heavy chewing force, clenching or bruxism can produce accelerated occlusal wear.

Detection

- Diagnosis is through periodic check up.
- In patients with bruxism and heavy occlusal forces, the check up should be planned more frequently than in others.
- Occlusal surface restored with metal may perforate over several years.

Treatment

- If the perforation is detected early before leakage or caries occurs, salvaging it with gold or amalgam restoration to seal the area may prolong its usefulness.
- When the metal surrounding the perforation is extremity thin, a new prosthesis should be fabricated.
- When a perforation exposes an amalgam core, simply leave the perforation untreated and examine it periodically.
- In porcelain restorations, wear of opposing enamel or metallic restoration is a matter of concern. The wear is faster in cases of heavy chewing forces, clenching or bruxism leading to pulp exposure. This often requires restoration of opposing teeth. Hence, in mouths where excessive wear is anticipated, it is better to restore occlusal surface with metal when opposing either tooth or metallic restorations.

4. Fracture of Tooth

Cause

- RCT treated teeth due to increasing brittleness.
- Around partial coverage retainers as a result of wear and increasing brittleness of tooth structure.
- Abutments of cantilever FPD due to excessive stress.
- Root fracture due to stress generated by dowel and core.[3]
- Periodontal disease of the abutment and mobility and resulting cantilever like situation leading to fracture of the anterior abutment.[4]
- Excessive tooth preparation, improper placement of pins, interfering occlusal contacts, trauma, heavy occlusal forces, forced placement of ill fitting prosthesis, trying to unseat a bridge incorrectly.

Detection

- Patient complaint of movement of the restoration or pain.
- Periodic clinical examination.
- Radiographs.

Treatment

- Use of cemented dowels as they are known to produce the least intraradicular stress.[3]
- If the fracture is minor creating only a small marginal defect and the restoration is adequately retained, the area may be filled with gold foil, amalgam or resin. This procedure adds some years of service to the restoration.
- Remove the prosthesis and evaluate the abutment. If it can be salvaged, plan a new prosthesis.
- If there is doubt about the prognosis, a new treatment needs to be planned in conjunction with periodontal and endodontic procedures.
- Rarely, in cases with multiple abutments, the fractured abutment can be dispensed with, the root is removed surgically and the retainer converted into a pontic.

5. Porcelain Fracture

Cause

- Improper design of the framework, e.g. sharp angles, irregular surface, extremely thin or perforated metal, incorrect placement of occlusal contacts.
- Improper choice of material.
- Poor handling and technique, e.g. incorporation of air bubbles, incorrect firing temperatures, repeated firing.
- Inadequate clearance during tooth preparation leading to inadequate thickness of all ceramic restoration.

Detection

- Patient complaint.
- Clinical examination.

Treatment

- The frequency of fractures has reduced with incorporation of new materials and techniques.
- Correction of etiology, e.g. proper diagnosis, correct tooth preparation, etc.
- If the failure occurs during normal function, shortly after the restoration is placed, the implication is that the conditions are not suitable for all ceramic restoration, and the replacement should be metal ceramic.

ESTHETIC FAILURES

1. Unacceptable Color Matching

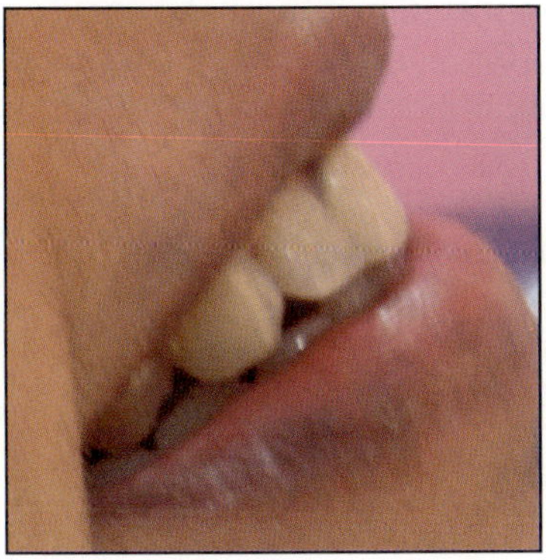

Fig. 16.3

Cause

Inadequate shade selection, inability to match the natural teeth with available porcelain colors, improper use of stains, metamerism, high esthetic demands of the patient, improper lighting of the operatory or even inadequate tooth reduction.

Treatment

- Modifications of preparation, repeat firing after proper shade selection, correct the lighting or use natural light, change the material.
- Over the years natural tooth may change color so the shade no longer matches. The situation might require a replacement of the restoration.

2. Display of Metal

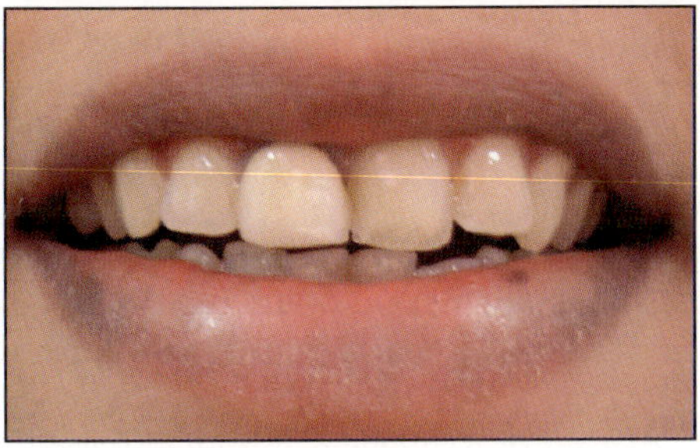

Fig. 16.4: Visible metal line along the margins

Cause

- Inadequate clearance for porcelain.
- Non-continuous layer of opaque.
- Display of metal in margins or the metal core.
- Partial coverage restorations extending to the facial surface or prepared in thin teeth leading to graying.

Treatment

- Use subgingival margins in esthetic areas.
- Proper selection of retainers.
- Proper porcelain manipulation techniques.
- Adequate clearance provided in tooth preparation.

3. Pontic Space Not Managed Adequately

Cause

- Pontic space available for a tooth may be larger due to movement of teeth or due to a pre-existing diastema.
- Pontic space may be lesser than normal due to tilting or drifting of teeth.
- The occluso- or inciso-gingival length of the pontic space may be greater due to loss of alveolar bone because of periodontal disease or trauma (Fig. 16.5).

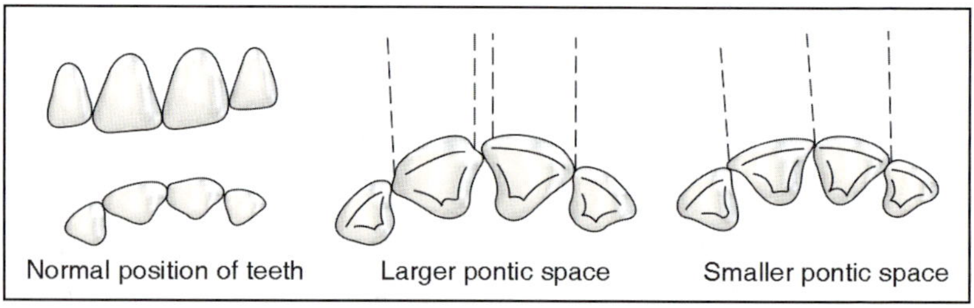

Fig. 16.5: Illusion of correct width by correct position of line angles

Treatment

- Adequate management of the pontic space by modification of pontic design. The technique is different for anterior and posterior regions and is discussed in the chapter on pontics.
- Orthodontic correction of teeth alignment before a prosthesis is fabricated.
- In mild cases, a distribution of space among abutments and pontics is a feasible option.

4. Poor Shape of Teeth

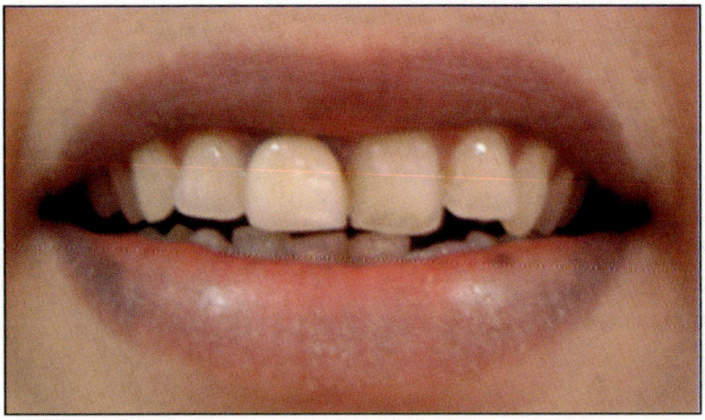

Fig. 16.6: Shape does not match with that of adjacent teeth

Cause

- Bulky restorations due to inadequate preparation to provide for proper porcelain thickness and manipulation to obtain proper shape.
- Improper cervical design of pontics with an artificial shadow on the ridge.

Treatment

- Provide proper clearance in preparation.
- The shape of the teeth should be designed in accordance with the patients teeth.

5. Diastema

Cause

- Retainers that do not contact adjacent teeth leave unaesthetic diastemata.
- A pre-existing diastema not adequately managed.

Treatment

- Proper choice and design of retainers.
- Adequate pontic space management.

6. Altered Soft Tissue Esthetics

Cause

- Inflammed soft tissues due to pontic impingement.
- Improper marginal fit and cervical form of the prosthesis that promote plaque accumulation and inflammation of soft tissues.

Treatment

- Contours and margin placement that promote soft tissue health.
- Point, pressureless contact of pontic on attached gingiva to promote health of edentulous ridge.[5]

7. Failure of Facings

Cause

- Dislodged facings.
- Fractured facings.
- Improper framework design or manipulation techniques.

Treatment

- Repair by recementation.
- Repair by overcasting to add a few years of service.
- Removal of the prosthesis and repeat using proper manipulation techniques.

PSYCHOLOGICAL FAILURE

Cause

High esthetic expectations of the patient.

Treatment

- Adequate education and treatment planning procedures should be followed even before the treatment is begun.
- All ceramic restorations should be considered in esthetic regions.
- Soft and hard tissue surgeries that can improve appearance should be employed.
- If an esthetic alternative is available with dental implants, it should be implemented.

CLASSIFICATION OF FPD FAILURES BY J.J. MANAPPALLIL[6]

He presented a classification based on the severity of the failure and conventional retreatment possibilities. He placed the conditions in 6 categories: Classes I to VI.

1. Class I Failures

i. Those that are correctable through occlusal adjustment or composite resin repairs without requiring replacement of the restoration.
ii. For example, loss of cement bond without any defects in preparation or casting. Correction may be done by recementation.

iii. Other class I problems may be correctable if the restoration is removed successfully.
iv. If removal attempts fail and the restoration has to be sectioned for removal or if the restoration or tooth is damaged during the attempt, the problem would be reclassified into a higher order of failure.

2. Class II Failures

- In a class II failure, the restoration itself is acceptable.
- However, the supporting tooth structure or foundation (core restoration, or post and core) requires repair or reconstruction.
- For example, loss of supporting tooth structure resulting from caries or fracture. Fractures that occur during attempts to remove a restoration also fall into class II.

3. Class III Failures

- Replacement of restoration is required with class III failures.
- However, the supporting tooth structure or foundation remains intact and would provide acceptable support for a replacement restoration.
- For example, unserviceable restorations due to defective margins, technical failures, or esthetic considerations.

4. Class IV Failures

- In class IV situations, the restoration requires replacement, and the supporting tooth structure or foundation is also deficient.
- Examples in this category include failures associated with caries, fracture of supporting tooth structure, or a defective foundation.
- Before making a new restoration, the tooth structure must be reinforced, reconstructed, or replaced.
- Various means can be used, including cores and post-and-core foundations.

5. Class V Failures

- In a class V failure, support structure can no longer provide adequate support for the existing restoration due to extensive fracture, carious destruction, periodontal problems, or other complications.
- A damaged tooth may require extraction.
- Even though the failure may involve tooth loss, restoration of the site is possible with conventional fixed prosthesis when other available teeth can be incorporated into a designed restoration.
- It also includes FPDs for which abutment teeth are not enough to provide adequate support. These abutment teeth can be treated and restored to function in a redesigned FPD, if additional abutment teeth are used to improve support.

6. Class VI Failures

- A class VI failure is the most severe failure.
- In this situation, a conventional fixed replacement is no longer possible. Supporting teeth have failed and there is lack of additional abutments for use in a redesigned restoration.
- An example of a class VI FPD failure would be the loss of the terminal abutment of an FPD replacing a first molar, assuming the third molar is missing or unsuitable for abutment service.
- Not all class VI failures are necessarily associated with loss of teeth.
- Examples would include failing long-span FPDs with supporting teeth that may be serviceable and are retained but they are not required to function as FPD abutments.
- In this situation, the treatment of choice would be to remove the pontic segments and restore the abutment teeth individually.
- Retreatment with a conventional FPD is no longer an option for a class VI failure.
- Other means of prosthodontic tooth replacement must be considered.

REFERENCES

1. Walton J.N., Gardner F.M., Agar J.R. A survey of crown and fixed partial denture failures: Length of service and reasons for replacement. *J Prosthet Dent* 1986;56:412–21.
2. Libby G., Arcuri M.R., LaVelle W.E., Hebl L. Longevity of fixed partial dentures. *J Prosthet Dent* 1997;78:127–31.
3. Goodacre C.J., Spolnik K.J. The prosthodontic management of endodontically treated tooth: A literature review. Part 1. Success and failure data, treatment concepts. *J Prosthodont* 1994;3:243–50.
4. Verrett R.G., Kaiser D.A. Fracture of a fixed partial denture abutment: A clinical report. *J Prosthet Dent* 2005;93:21–3.
5. Brehm T.W. Diagnosis and treatment planning for fixed prosthodontics. *J Prosthet Dent* 1973;30:876–81.
6. Manappallil J.J. Classification system for conventional crown and fixed partial denture failures. *J Prosthet Dent* 2008;99:293–8.

Index

Reader's Note

Reader's Note

Reader's Note

Reader's Note